PUBLIC HEALTH IN THE 21ST CENTURY

INFLUENZA: PANDEMIC LESSONS AND VACCINE EFFORTS

PUBLIC HEALTH IN THE 21ST CENTURY

Additional books in this series can be found on Nova's website under the Series tab.

Additional E-books in this series can be found on Nova's website under the E-books tab.

PUBLIC HEALTH IN THE 21ST CENTURY

INFLUENZA: PANDEMIC LESSONS AND VACCINE EFFORTS

RICHARD A. COLON
EDITOR

Nova Science Publishers, Inc.
New York

For permission to use material from this book please contact us:
Telephone 631-231-7269; Fax 631-231-8175
Web Site: http://www.novapublishers.com

Library of Congress Cataloging-in-Publication Data

ISBN 978-1-62100-174-4

Published by Nova Science Publishers, Inc. † New York

CONTENTS

PREFACE

This book examines federal funding from fiscal year 2005 through March 2011 for alternative technologies and the status of manufacturers' efforts; challenges to development and licensure identified by stakeholders and how HHS is addressing those challenges.

Chapter 1 The 2009 H1N1 influenza pandemic was the first human pandemic in over four decades, and the Centers for Disease Control and Prevention (CDC) estimate that there were as many as 89 million U.S. cases. Over $6 billion was available for the response, led by the Departments of Health and Human Services (HHS) and Homeland Security (DHS), with coordination provided by the Homeland Security Council (HSC) through its National Security Staff (NSS). In particular, HHS's CDC worked with states and localities to communicate with the public and to distribute H1N1 vaccine and supplies.

GAO was asked (1) how HHS used the funding, (2) the key issues raised by the federal response, and (3) the actions taken to identify and incorporate lessons learned. GAO reviewed documents and interviewed officials from five states about their interaction with the federal government. GAO also reviewed documents and interviewed officials from HHS, DHS, the Department of Labor's Occupational Safety and Health Administration (OSHA), NSS, and others, such as associations.

Chapter 2- Production delays for the 2009 H1N1 pandemic vaccine using the current egg-based production technology heightened interest in alternative technologies that could expand the supply or accelerate the availability of influenza vaccine. Within the federal government, the Department of Health and Human Services (HHS) and the Department of Defense (DOD) support the development of technologies that can be used in producing influenza vaccines. HHS's Food and Drug Administration (FDA) reviews licensing applications for new vaccine, and the Department of State is the U.S. diplomatic liaison to the international entity that declares worldwide pandemics.

GAO was asked to review federal activities for the development of alternative technologies used in producing influenza vaccine. This report examines (1) federal funding from fiscal year 2005 through March 2011 for alternative technologies and the status of manufacturers' efforts, (2) challenges to development and licensure identified by stakeholders, and (3) how HHS is addressing those challenges.

GAO reviewed HHS and DOD documents and funding data. GAO also interviewed stakeholders, including manufacturer representatives, industry associations, and other experts on challenges to development and licensure. GAO interviewed HHS officials on how they are addressing those challenges.

In: Influenza
Editor: Richard A. Colon
ISBN: 978-1-62100-174-4

Chapter 1

INFLUENZA PANDEMIC: LESSONS FROM THE H1N1 PANDEMIC SHOULD BE INCORPORATED INTO FUTURE PLANNING*

United States Government Accountability Office

WHY GAO DID THIS STUDY

The 2009 H1N1 influenza pandemic was the first human pandemic in over four decades, and the Centers for Disease Control and Prevention (CDC) estimate that there were as many as 89 million U.S. cases. Over $6 billion was available for the response, led by the Departments of Health and Human Services (HHS) and Homeland Security (DHS), with coordination provided by the Homeland Security Council (HSC) through its National Security Staff (NSS). In particular, HHS's CDC worked with states and localities to communicate with the public and to distribute H1N1 vaccine and supplies.

GAO was asked (1) how HHS used the funding, (2) the key issues raised by the federal response, and (3) the actions taken to identify and incorporate lessons learned. GAO reviewed documents and interviewed officials from five states about their interaction with the federal government. GAO also reviewed documents and interviewed officials from HHS, DHS, the Department of

* This is an edited, reformatted and augmented version of a United States Government Accountability Office GAO-11-632 publication, dated June 2011.

Labor's Occupational Safety and Health Administration (OSHA), NSS, and others, such as associations.

WHAT GAO RECOMMENDS

GAO recommends that the HSC direct the NSS, in concert with HHS and DHS, to incorporate lessons from the H1N1 pandemic into future planning and share these lessons with key stakeholders. NSS agreed to take the recommendations under advisement. HHS, DHS, and OSHA provided comments and generally agreed with our findings.

WHAT GAO FOUND

As of December 2010, HHS had spent about two-thirds of the $6.15 billion that it had available for the H1N1 pandemic response. HHS spent the majority of the funds on developing and purchasing H1N1 vaccine and providing grants to all the states and selected local jurisdictions. State and local health officials reported that the grant funding was critical to their response efforts but also noted challenges presented by the grants' administrative requirements. HHS's spending plans for the remaining $1.98 billion include longer-term pandemic preparation efforts, such as activities to reduce the length of time required to produce a vaccine.

Several key issues were raised by the federal government's response to the H1N1 pandemic.

- Prior pandemic planning efforts and federal funding paid off, although specific aspects of prior planning were not relied on because of the nature of the H1N1 pandemic. For example, interagency meetings and exercises built relationships that were valuable during the response. Prior funding built capacity in several areas, including vaccine production.
- The credibility of all levels of government was diminished when the amount of vaccine available to the public in October 2009 did not meet expectations set by federal officials. However, state and local jurisdictions valued the flexibility that they had in deciding their distribution methods. Additionally, while the use of a central distributor

for the vaccines was generally cited as an effective practice, the 100-dose minimum order was viewed to be problematic.

- Public surveys generally found CDC's communication efforts to be successful in reaching a range of audiences; however, these messages fell short in meeting the needs of some non-English-speaking populations.
- Deployment of the Strategic National Stockpile—a supply of medicines and medical supplies to be used for a national emergency—met the established goal. However, CDC and state officials identified gaps in planning, including disparities between the materials expected and those delivered, as well as the need for long-term storage plans for stockpile materials.

The NSS asked federal agencies—including HHS and DHS—to complete after-action reports based on their involvement in the pandemic response. The NSS has not determined if these reports—and the associated lessons learned—will be shared with key stakeholders. Nevertheless, a DHS official commented that sharing lessons from the reports with key stakeholders would foster a spirit of government transparency and might help build stakeholder trust.

ABBREVIATIONS

ACIP	Advisory Committee on Immunization Practices
ASPR	Office of the Assistant Secretary for Preparedness and Response
ASTHO	Association of State and Territorial Health Officials
BARDA	Biomedical Advanced Research and Development Authority
CDC	Centers for Disease Control and Prevention
DHS	Department of Homeland Security
EUA	emergency use authorization
FDA	Food and Drug Administration
HHS	Department of Health and Human Services
HSC	Homeland Security Council
IOM	Institute of Medicine
NACCHO	National Association of County and City Health Officials
NSS	National Security Staff
OSHA	Occupational Safety and Health Administration
PHER	Public Health Emergency Response

SNS	Strategic National Stockpile
WHO	World Health Organization

June 27, 2011

The Honorable Fred Upton
Chairman

The Honorable Henry A. Waxman
Ranking Member
Committee on Energy and Commerce
House of Representatives

The Honorable Bennie G. Thompson
Ranking Member
Committee on Homeland Security
House of Representatives

The Honorable Roy Blunt
United States Senate

The Honorable Joe Barton
House of Representatives

In Response To The Global Spread Of The H1N1 Influenza Virus, The United Nations' World Health Organization (WHO)[1] Declared The First Human Influenza Pandemic In More Than Four Decades On June 11, 2009.[2] Prior To This Declaration, H1N1 Influenza Had Spread Across The United States After First Being Detected In California In April 2009.[3] The Department Of Health And Human Services' (HHS) Centers For Disease Control And Prevention (CDC) Estimated That There Were As Many As 89 Million U.S. Cases Of H1N1 influenza from April 2009 to April 2010.[4] CDC estimated that these cases led to as many as 403,000 hospitalizations and 18,300 deaths during that period, with a disproportionate number of children affected as compared to typical influenza seasons. WHO declared that the 2009 H1N1 influenza pandemic ended on August 10, 2010.

Prior to the H1N1 pandemic, federal, state, and local governments were involved in national pandemic planning and preparedness activities. At the federal level these activities—which were largely coordinated by the Homeland

Security Council (HSC)[5]—included releasing a national pandemic strategy and a national pandemic implementation plan in 2005 and 2006, respectively, and holding regular interagency meetings. Additionally, as part of pandemic planning, HHS funded the development of medical countermeasures, such as vaccines and antiviral drugs.[6] The national pandemic strategy and the national pandemic implementation plan designated HHS and the Department of Homeland Security (DHS) as the two agencies that would lead a federal response to an influenza pandemic. However, because these planning and preparedness activities were geared toward responding to an avian influenza pandemic that originated overseas and had a higher fatality rate, some adjustments during the H1N1 pandemic response were necessary. Accordingly, the National Security Staff (NSS), which supports the HSC, developed an additional document, the *National Framework for 2009-H1N1 Influenza Preparedness and Response*.[7]

To aid in the response to the H1N1 pandemic, the federal government took a variety of measures. The Congress appropriated funds to HHS specifically to prepare for and respond to an influenza pandemic as part of a supplemental appropriation in June 2009.[8] The federal government—and particularly CDC—collaborated with state and local jurisdictions,[9] professional associations, and private health care providers, among others, to take a variety of measures to mitigate the spread of disease, such as communicating with the public, distributing vaccines, conducting surveillance, and distributing items from the Strategic National Stockpile (SNS).[10]

Because of the possibility of another influenza pandemic and our prior work on pandemic preparedness,[11] you asked us to examine the lessons learned from the federal response to the H1N1 pandemic and identify how the federal government is incorporating these lessons into future pandemic planning. As agreed, this report examines (1) how HHS used 2009 supplemental funding to respond to the H1N1 pandemic, (2) the key issues raised by the federal government's response to the H1N1 pandemic, and (3) the actions that federal agencies are taking to identify and incorporate lessons learned from the issues that arose from the H1N1 pandemic into planning.

To examine how HHS used the 2009 supplemental funding to respond to the H1N1 pandemic, we reviewed the Supplemental Appropriations Act, 2009; HHS's reports to the Congress detailing the ways that HHS spent funds; and HHS's amended spending plans that were also submitted to the Congress.[12] To determine the reliability of the data in these reports, we reviewed the reports for internal consistency and resolved questions with appropriate HHS officials; we did not independently verify the information provided in these reports. We believe that the data are sufficiently reliable for our purposes. While HHS used funds from other appropriations in the H1N1 pandemic response effort, we focused our review on the $6.15 billion available to HHS that was provided through the 2009 supplemental appropriation. Because this appropriation required that a portion of the supplemental funds be directed toward upgrading state and local public health capacity, we reviewed requirements of the grants that were awarded to state and local jurisdictions for this purpose. To examine how state and local jurisdictions used the grant funds, we reviewed documents and interviewed officials from CDC's Division of State and Local Readiness, the Association of State and Territorial Health Officials (ASTHO), and the National Association of County and City Health Officials (NACCHO). We also interviewed officials involved in the H1N1 pandemic response in a sample of five states—Georgia, Nebraska, Texas, Vermont, and Washington—to learn about how their jurisdictions used the response funds. We chose these states to provide insight into the experiences of a range of states; however, their experiences are not generalizable to all 50 states. We selected states that reflected a range of key characteristics, including when the state first reported experiencing widespread H1N1 influenza activity, interim state-specific H1N1 vaccination rates among the initial target groups for the H1N1 vaccine, population in 2008, census region, total grant amount awarded to the state for the H1N1 pandemic response, and the state's public health structure. Appendix I includes information on the five selected states. In general, within each state, we spoke with officials from the governor's office, the state health agency, the state emergency management agency, and the state education agency.[13] In addition, to provide an example of how the territories and insular areas used pandemic grant funds, we contacted officials from the U.S. Virgin Islands based on the same criteria that we used to select the states in our sample.

To examine the key issues raised by the federal government's response to the H1N1 pandemic, we focused on the actions of HHS and DHS because they share federal leadership responsibilities for pandemic influenza response. Within HHS, we reviewed documents and interviewed officials from the Office of the Assistant Secretary for Preparedness and Response (ASPR), ASPR's Biomedical Advanced Research and Development Authority (BARDA), the Food and Drug Administration (FDA), and CDC. Within DHS, we reviewed documents and interviewed officials from the Office of Health Affairs, Directorate for Management, Office of Operations Coordination, and Federal Emergency Management Agency. Because of their respective roles in the H1N1 pandemic response, we also reviewed documents and interviewed officials from the Department of Education's (Education) Office of Safe and Drug Free Schools regarding school closure policies and the Department of Labor's Occupational

Safety and Health Administration (OSHA) regarding guidance on the use of personal protective equipment and the protection of workers' safety and health.[14] To learn about the federal government's interaction with state and local jurisdictions, we interviewed officials from the same judgmental sample of five states. We also reviewed reports and interviewed officials from the U.S. Virgin Islands, ASTHO, NACCHO, the National Governors Association, the Center for Infectious Disease Research and Policy, the Association of Immunization Managers, the Institute of Medicine (IOM), and the National Indian Health Board.[15]

To examine the actions that federal agencies are taking to identify and incorporate lessons learned from the issues that arose from the H1N1 pandemic into planning, we interviewed officials and reviewed documents from HHS, DHS, Education, and the Department of Labor. We interviewed officials from the NSS, which was responsible for developing the *National Framework for 2009-H1N1 Influenza Preparedness Response* and for holding interagency coordination meetings during the H1N1 pandemic response. We also examined the *National Response Framework*—a guide for the federal government to use in responding to domestic incidents— which specifies that evaluation and continual process improvement are cornerstones of effective preparedness. The framework notes that improvement planning should develop specific recommendations for changes in practice, timelines for implementation, and assignments for completion.[16]

We conducted this performance audit from April 2010 to June 2011 in accordance with generally accepted government auditing standards. Those standards require that we plan and perform the audit to obtain sufficient, appropriate evidence to provide a reasonable basis for our findings and conclusions based on our audit objectives. We believe that the evidence obtained provides a reasonable basis for our findings and conclusions based on our audit objectives.

BACKGROUND

Pandemic Preparedness Prior to the H1N1 Pandemic

The emergence of H5N1 avian influenza (also known as avian influenza or bird flu) in Asia in 2003 raised concerns among experts that it or another influenza virus might significantly mutate, resulting in a human influenza pandemic. This led to the development of the national pandemic strategy and national pandemic implementation plan.[17] This strategy and plan established that the Secretary of Health and Human Services is to lead the federal public health and medical response to a pandemic and the Secretary of Homeland Security is to lead the overall domestic incident management and federal coordination.

Additionally, prior to the H1N1 pandemic, the Congress appropriated funds to support the federal government's influenza pandemic preparedness and improve related state and local public health capabilities. In fiscal year 2006, the Congress appropriated about $5.60 billion to HHS through supplemental appropriations to support pandemic preparedness and response efforts, such as vaccine and antiviral drug development and stockpiling, state and local preparedness, and international collaboration.[18] HHS reported spending more than half of the funds (about $3.10 billion) on activities related to vaccine development, stockpiling, and infrastructure improvement. For example, the department awarded contracts to two domestic influenza vaccine manufacturers to retrofit their facilities—that is, to upgrade existing facilities to optimize and enhance their ability to produce influenza vaccines. HHS spent nearly a quarter of the funds (about $1.30 billion) on activities related to developing and stockpiling antiviral drugs. For example, the department completed the purchase of 50 million courses of antiviral drugs for the SNS and provided funding to states to increase state stockpiles as part of its goal of ensuring the availability of antiviral drug treatment courses for 25 percent of the U.S. population in case of an influenza pandemic.[19] HHS invested in the development of Peramivir, an intravenously administered antiviral drug for seriously ill patients with influenza. HHS also funded the development and clinical trials of influenza diagnostic testing devices that allow for the diagnosis of influenza in a variety of settings.[20]

2009 H1N1 Pandemic

The first case of H1N1 influenza was detected in the United States on April 15, 2009. Cases of H1N1 influenza first appeared in California and Texas, and soon spread across the country and around the world. (See fig. 1 for a timeline of key events.) At the same time, an outbreak of H1N1 influenza was occurring in Mexico. In response, the NSS developed the *National Framework for 2009-H1N1 Influenza Preparedness and Response* as a tool to guide the federal response efforts.[21] The framework was built on the existing national pandemic strategy and national pandemic implementation plan and contained four pillars for the response: surveillance, mitigation measures, vaccination, and communication and education.

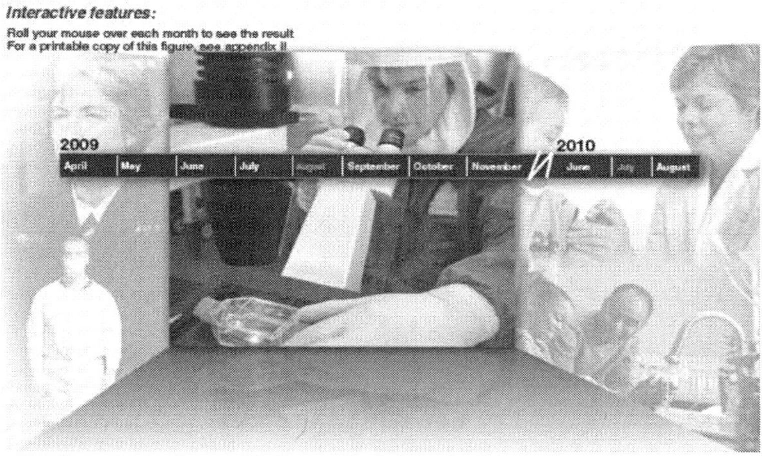

Sources: GAO analysis; James Gathany, Cade Martin (photos).

Notes: The declaration of a public health emergency, pursuant to 42 U.S.C. § 247d, provided the basis for the Secretary of Health and Human Services to exercise the authority under certain circumstances to approve the emergency use of unapproved drugs, devices, or biological products (or the emergency use of approved drugs, devices, or biological products for unapproved uses) through emergency use authorizations. 21 U.S.C. § 360bbb-3.

The President's declaration of a national emergency pursuant to the National Emergencies Act provided the Secretary of Health and Human Services the authority to temporarily waive or modify certain requirements affecting the health care system throughout the duration of the public health emergency. 50 U.S.C. §§ 1621 and 1631; 42 U.S.C. § 1320b-5.

The release of 25 percent of the influenza supplies from the Strategic National Stockpile included antiviral drugs and equipment to protect against influenza transmission, such as face masks, respirators, gowns, and gloves.

Figure 1. Key Events Related to the H1N1 Influenza Pandemic in the United States, April 2009 through August 2010.

The H1N1 pandemic occurred in two waves in the United States.[22] The first wave occurred during spring 2009 and the second wave during fall 2009, with H1N1 influenza activity peaking in October 2009, based on the number of new cases. A greater proportion of children and young adults, as well as pregnant women, were adversely affected by the H1N1 influenza virus as compared to the typical influenza season.

H1N1 Vaccine Production and Distribution

When the H1N1 influenza outbreak occurred in April 2009, HHS began working to isolate the H1N1 influenza strain and worked with five vaccine manufacturers to develop a 2009 H1N1 influenza vaccine (H1N1 vaccine) to protect the public against H1N1 influenza.[23] The H1N1 vaccines were manufactured using the same methods that these manufacturers used for seasonal influenza vaccine production.

In anticipation of the availability of the H1N1 vaccine and the possibility that initial supply might not meet demand for the vaccine, in July 2009, CDC's Advisory Committee on Immunization Practices (ACIP) issued recommendations for the target groups for the H1N1 vaccine.[24] These five target groups, comprising about 159 million persons, were recommended to be first to receive the H1N1 vaccine.[25] ACIP also identified a subset of the initial target groups, comprising about 42 million persons, to whom providers should give priority if H1N1 vaccine availability was too limited to initiate vaccination for all people in the five initial target groups.[26] However, at the time it made the recommendations, ACIP did not predict that there would be a need to limit vaccine to the subset of the target groups in most areas of the country.

Unlike seasonal influenza vaccine, which is largely purchased by the private sector, the federal government purchased all of the H1N1 vaccine licensed for use in the United States. HHS allocated doses to each state for distribution based on the overall population of the state. The states, in turn, placed orders for their allocated doses and determined which providers should receive the vaccine. CDC estimated that from October 2009 through May 2010, 27 percent of the U.S. population over the age of 6 months (about 81 million people) was vaccinated against H1N1 influenza, including about 34 percent of individuals in the initial target groups.[27]

Strategic National Stockpile

In addition to the production and distribution of the H1N1 vaccine, another federal action in response to the H1N1 pandemic was the deployment of influenza response supplies from the SNS. The SNS, managed by CDC, contains large quantities of medicine and medical supplies intended to protect and treat the public if there is a public health emergency that is severe enough that local supplies may be exhausted. Each state has plans to receive materials from the SNS and distribute them to local communities as quickly as possible. The H1N1 pandemic marked the largest deployment of materials from the SNS to date in an emergency situation, according to CDC.

HHS FUNDED A RANGE OF PANDEMIC INFLUENZA ACTIVITIES WITH SUPPLEMENTAL FUNDS

Most Supplemental Funds Were Spent on Vaccine Purchase and Support of State and Local Pandemic Response Efforts

The Congress Appropriated Funds to HHS to Meet the Threat of Pandemic Influenza

HHS had $6.15 billion available from the 2009 supplemental appropriation to spend on pandemic influenza activities. Specifically, the Congress appropriated $1.85 billion immediately to HHS in June 2009, shortly after WHO declared the start of the pandemic. The Congress also appropriated up to $5.80 billion in additional contingent funding. These contingent funds would only be available in the amounts designated by the President, in written notices to the Congress, as emergency funds required to address critical needs related to emerging influenza viruses. In July and September of 2009, the President notified the Congress of the need for additional funding, and accordingly, $4.54 billion of the contingent funds became available to HHS. From this $4.54 billion, HHS transferred about $241 million to other departments, which left about $4.30 billion available for HHS.[28] As of December 2010, the remaining $1.259 billion from the contingent fund was not designated by the President as required to address critical needs related to emerging influenza viruses; however, these funds were rescinded under the fiscal year 2011 continuing appropriations act.[29]

HHS Has Spent Almost 70 Percent of Available Supplemental Funds

From June 2009 through December 2010, HHS spent about $4.17 billion (about two-thirds)[30] of the $6.15 billion that it had available from the 2009 supplemental appropriation, according to HHS's report to the Congress on pandemic influenza preparedness spending.[31] Of the $4.17 billion spent by HHS, about $1.72 billion (41 percent) was spent on vaccine production, which includes the purchase of H1N1 vaccine from five influenza vaccine manufacturers, adjuvants,[32] and ancillary supplies, such as needles and syringes, distributed along with the H1N1 vaccine. Specifically, HHS funded the development of and purchased over 190 million doses of the H1N1 vaccine and purchased 200 million ancillary supply kits.[33]

Of the $4.17 billion spent by HHS, about $1.49 billion (36 percent) was spent on supporting state and local jurisdictions' response to the H1N1 pandemic. The majority of these funds were provided to the states through Public Health Emergency Response (PHER) grants.[34]

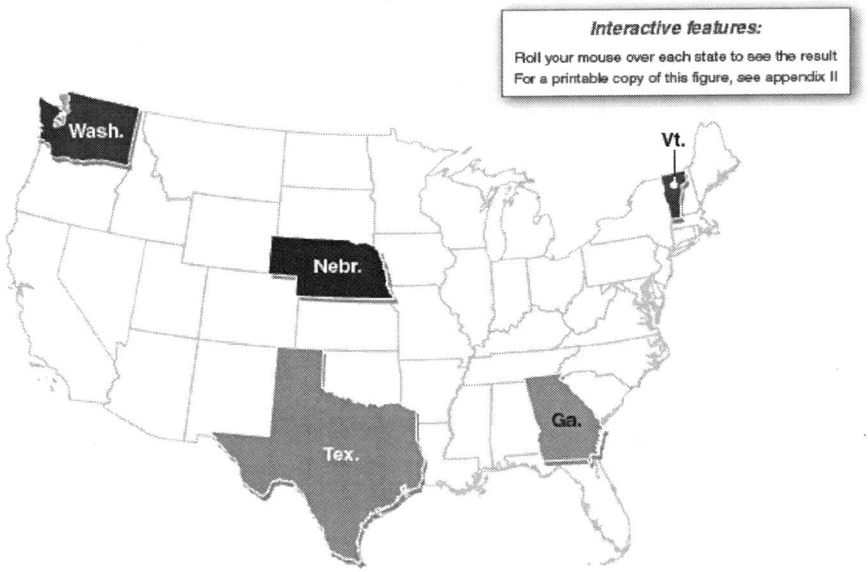

Sources: GAO analysis of state data; Map Resources (map).

Figure 2. Examples of Ways That State and Local Jurisdictions Used the PHER Grants.

The PHER grant funds were distributed in four phases beginning in August 2009, with each phase of funding targeting specific focus areas, such as vaccination or communication efforts with high-risk populations.[35] A report by ASTHO concluded that state and local jurisdictions could not have responded as effectively to the H1N1 pandemic without the PHER grant funds, particularly given the ongoing budgetary constraints of states.[36] (See fig. 2 for examples of how states and local jurisdictions used the PHER grants.) HHS spent the remaining $1 billion (24 percent) on other purposes. See table 1 for information on HHS activities supported by the 2009 supplemental appropriation.

Table 1. HHS Activities Supported by the 2009 Supplemental Appropriation

Activity	Amount spent as of December 31, 2010 (in millions)	Percentage of total funds spent
Vaccine production includes purchase of H1N1 vaccine, adjuvant,a and ancillary supplies for the H1N1 vaccine.	$1,719	41.3
PHER grants includes grants to state and local jurisdictions to upgrade state and local public health capacity.	1,404	33.7
CDC vaccination campaign includes contracts to support the distribution of H1N1 vaccine and ancillary supplies, H1N1 vaccine safety and effectiveness monitoring, and a communications campaign on vaccination and prevention.	340	8.2
Antiviral drugs includes the purchase of pediatric doses of antiviral drugs in response to the disproportionate effects of H1N1 influenza on children.	231	5.6
CDC domestic response includes funds for deployment of CDC staff to support investigations into the H1N1 outbreak along the borders and in the United States and production and distribution of a diagnostic test kit for H1N1 influenza.	199	4.8
Ongoing H1N1 activities includes funds to continue development of intravenous presentations of an antiviral drug for persons with influenza and a program to monitor the effects of use of H1N1 vaccine and antiviral drugs by pregnant women and the babies they bore.	95	2.3
Hospital Preparedness Program includes grants through states to hospitals for health care workforce protection and the development of plans to optimize usage of the health care system during an influenza pandemic.	90	2.2
CDC international response includes support for H1N1 influenza surveillance, laboratory and research projects in over 13 countries, and personnel support provided to WHO regional offices to handle H1N1 pandemic surge activities.	44	1.1
CDC communications includes funds for consumer behavioral research on messaging; use of a Web-based media monitoring system to assess message dissemination by the media about H1N1 influenza; support of pandemic influenza tabletop exercises involving national, regional, and local media outlets; and translation of pandemic influenza materials into various languages.	31	0.7
Countermeasureb development and regulation at FDA includes the development, evaluation, licensure, and safety monitoring of the H1N1 vaccine, and FDA activities to facilitate the availability and safety monitoring of H1N1 diagnostic tests, personal protective equipment, and antiviral drugs.	9	0.2
Compensation includes funds used to support the administration of the Countermeasures Injury Compensation Program, which will provide compensation to individuals with injuries caused by certain countermeasures administered to diagnose, mitigate, prevent, or treat harm from specified material threats.c	4	0.1
ASPR deployment/operations support includes costs associated with sending ASPR staff to states and territories during the H1N1 pandemic.	1	0.0
Total	$4,167	100.0

Table 1.Continued

Source: GAO analysis of HHS data.

Notes: Numbers may not sum to totals because of rounding. The information presented in this table is based on Department of Health and Human Services, Report to Congress: December 2010 Report, Pandemic Influenza Preparedness Spending (Washington, D.C., February 2011). HHS is submitting biannual reports to the Congress on the 2009 supplemental appropriation. The February 2011 report covers spending through December 2010.

HHS reported that it transferred $241 million to the Departments of Defense, Veterans Affairs, State, and Agriculture. Since HHS spent the majority of the 2009 supplemental appropriation, we did not determine how the $241.20 million transferred to these other departments was spent by them. We did not independently verify the amount that was transferred. The 2009 supplemental appropriation requires that all funds transferred to these departments go toward purposes related to preparing for or responding to an influenza pandemic.

[a] Adjuvants are substances that may be added to a vaccine to increase the body's immune response. While adjuvants were purchased by HHS as a precautionary measure, they were not used in the H1N1 vaccine.

[b] Medical countermeasures are medications, biological products, or devices that treat, identify, or prevent harm from a biological or other agent that may cause a public health emergency. Medical countermeasures for use during an influenza pandemic may include vaccines, antiviral drugs, personal respirators, and influenza diagnostic tests.

[c] The Countermeasures Injury Compensation Program, administered by HHS's Health Resources and Services Administration, provides compensation for medical expenses, lost employment income, and/or death benefits for eligible individuals injured as a result of receiving certain countermeasures, such as vaccines, antiviral drugs, diagnostic tests, and personal protective equipment.

States Experienced Challenges with Grant Administration During the Pandemic Response

While the PHER grants were critical to state and local jurisdictions, officials from state and local jurisdictions reported experiencing challenges with the administrative requirements of the PHER grants.

- ASTHO reported that state officials found the need to submit multiple applications for the various phases of the grant, and the time spent waiting for approvals, to be time consuming during the response. Additionally, the different limitations on the use of funds in each phase made it difficult for states to plan and manage their response activities.[37]
- Some of the local officials we interviewed reported that the specific spending requirements of the PHER funding were heavily weighted toward vaccination activities and that funds were neither flexible nor sufficient enough to address epidemiology and laboratory expenses.[38] Officials from Washington's Department of Health, for example, echoed

this concern and told us that some local health jurisdictions in the state did not have enough funding for surveillance and laboratory expenses, but had more than enough designated for vaccination activities. Almost half of states applied for the last phase of funding— and 15 states received the funds—which were available in early 2010 for targeting special, hard-to-reach populations for vaccination. In most cases, the states were not eligible for these funds because they had sufficient funds left over from the previous three phases to conduct vaccination outreach to hard-to-reach, high-risk populations.

CDC officials who worked on the PHER grant program said they were aware of the challenges that states faced with the grant process and were working on addressing some of these challenges in preparation for the next public health emergency. To reduce the time that it takes for funding to reach the states, CDC officials identified ways to save time for various procedures, such as preparing draft grant guidance in advance of public health emergencies. Additionally, CDC officials told us that they are working with ASTHO to help states be better prepared to quickly use federal funding that might become available in an emergency situation. For example, CDC officials noted that states with independent local health jurisdictions could establish draft contracts with these local health jurisdictions so that funding could flow more quickly down to the local level. In addition to these measures, CDC officials are working with their General Counsel's office to look at any authorities that they may have to move funds through existing cooperative agreements in an emergency. CDC officials also agreed that the phases of the PHER grants were heavily weighted toward vaccination, but noted that they made that decision because of the anticipation that the vaccination campaign would be the largest component of the public health response. In August 2010, the state and local jurisdictions received a no-cost extension that allows them to spend the PHER grant funds through July 2011. CDC expects to have detailed data regarding the ways that states spent these funds after the grant program expires.

HHS Plans for Remaining Supplemental Funds Include Efforts to Prepare For Future Pandemics

When WHO declared the H1N1 pandemic over in August 2010, HHS had not spent about $1.98 billion of the 2009 supplemental funds. Plans for the remaining funds include efforts that HHS identified to prepare for future pandemics. (See table 2 for additional information on how HHS plans to use these funds.) These longer-term preparations were primarily identified by an HHS review of public health emergency medical countermeasures.[39] This review found, for example, that continued, long-term investment is needed to improve domestic influenza vaccine production capacity and to shorten the amount of time needed to produce an influenza vaccine during a pandemic. According to HHS's August 2010 amended spending plan, a portion of the remaining funds will be spent on efforts to reduce the length of time required to produce a pandemic vaccine.[40] Specifically, HHS planned to spend $431 million—or 22 percent of these funds—on the development of new influenza vaccine technologies. Further, about $50 million (3 percent) is planned for enhancing the available domestic fill and finish capacity—the final stage in the vaccine production process that places the vaccine in the appropriate delivery device—which has been cited as a bottleneck in the existing influenza vaccine production process.

Table 2. HHS's Planned Spending for Remaining Influenza Pandemic Funds from the 2009 Supplemental Appropriation, as of December 31, 2010

Primary activity	Subactivity	Amount (in millions)
Influenza vaccine production		$758
	New vaccine production technologies includes supporting the development of new influenza vaccine technologies that would shorten vaccine production time.	431
	Centers for Innovation in Advanced Development and Manufacturing includes the support of multiuse facilities that could be used to expand influenza vaccine production capacity during a pandemic.	108
	H5N1 prepandemic vaccine storage and stability testing includes activities to enlarge the H5N1 prepandemic vaccine and antiviral drug stockpiles and conduct stability testing to determine the vaccine's shelf life.	54
	Adjuvants[a] includes support for clinical tests of existing and new vaccines with adjuvants, development of regulatory guidance for adjuvants, and further research and development.	60
	Domestic fill and finish manufacturing network includes activities to develop a network of facilities with sufficient capacity to rapidly fill the vials, syringes, and sprayers required for delivery of influenza vaccine during a pandemic.	50

Table 2.Continued

	Influenza vaccine potency and sterility test development includes activities to develop methods to improve and shorten the time needed for vaccine potency tests that determine the amount of antigen in a vaccine and sterility tests that ensure that a vaccine is not contaminated.[b]	30
	Vaccine seed optimization includes support of activities that would hasten and standardize the process for generating the virus strains used to manufacture influenza vaccines.	24
	H1N1 vaccine recovery project includes H1N1 vaccine storage and disposal.	1
	Egg supply includes support for a year-round egg supply that could be used to develop an influenza vaccine in a pandemic.[c]	1
Antiviral drugs	Antiviral drug advanced development includes funding for advanced development of Peramivir, an intravenously administered antiviral drug that was used during the H1N1 pandemic, plus other development activities at HHS.	435
Advanced development of diagnostics	Advanced development of diagnostic testing devices for influenza	76
HHS/CDC		623
	CDC replenishment of supplies in the SNS includes supplies that are needed during an influenza pandemic.	257
	CDC base influenza activities supports a portion of CDC's fiscal year 2011 SNS and influenza activities.	225
	HHS/CDC Surveillance, Lab Capacity and Communications Activities supports the continuation and completion of activities begun in response to the H1N1 pandemic. This includes measures such as virus detection and countermeasure development.	141
National Institutes of Health	Pandemic influenza–related research activities	33
Compensation	Countermeasures Injury Compensation Program, which provides compensation for eligible individuals injured as a result of receiving certain medical countermeasures.	58
Total		$1,983

Source: GAO analysis of HHS data.

Notes: Totals may not sum to totals because of rounding. The information presented in this table is based in part on Department of Health and Human Services, Report to Congress: December 2010 Report, Pandemic Influenza Preparedness Spending (Washington, D.C., February 2011), and Department of Health and Human Services, Amended Spending Plan for 2009 Supplemental Funding, as reported to the Congress in August 2010.

[a] Adjuvants are substances that may be added to a vaccine to increase the body's immune response.

[b] An antigen is the active substance in a vaccine that provides immunity by causing the body to produce protective antibodies to fight off a particular influenza strain.

[c] Current influenza vaccines are prepared from materials grown in chicken eggs.

FEDERAL RESPONSE TO THE H1N1 PANDEMICHIGHLIGHTED A NUMBER OF KEY ISSUES

Several key issues were raised by the federal government's response to the H1N1 pandemic. These relate to

- prior planning and funding,
- availability of vaccine and related plans for distribution,
- public communication, and
- the SNS.

Not All Aspects of the Existing Strategy and Plan Were Relied on, but Earlier Funding and Planning Paid off

Elements of National Pandemic Strategy and Implementation Plan Were Not Relied on Because of the Nature of the H1N1 Pandemic

Given the specific characteristics of the H1N1 pandemic, the federal government did not rely on some aspects of the national pandemic strategy and national pandemic implementation plan, such as critical infrastructure protection and border and trade measures. The national pandemic strategy and national pandemic implementation plan were based on a scenario of a severe 1918-like pandemic, as well as the existing threat that an avian influenza strain, originating overseas, would cause the next pandemic. During the early months of the H1N1 outbreak, officials from DHS and other departments reported that the action items in the national pandemic implementation plan for which their respective departments had responsibility—such as border and trade measures— were not relevant for the H1N1 outbreak, and therefore were not activated.[41] Federal officials noted, however, that while these actions were not taken in the H1N1 pandemic response, they could be important in a future pandemic with different characteristics, such as if there is a severe pandemic that affects critical infrastructure.[42]

Another aspect of the national pandemic strategy and national pandemic implementation plan that was not fully tested was the shared leadership roles and responsibilities for both HHS and DHS in responding to an influenza pandemic. We previously reported that it was unclear how this shared leadership would work in practice. Under the national pandemic strategy and national pandemic implementation plan, both departments share leadership responsibilities—HHS to manage the federal public health and medical response and DHS to lead domestic incident management and federal coordination. As a result, we recommended that HHS and DHS work together to develop and conduct rigorous testing, training, and exercising for pandemic influenza to ensure that the federal leadership roles are clearly defined and understood and that leaders are able to effectively execute shared responsibilities.[43] HHS officials told us that they are planning to exercise these roles with DHS.

The shared leadership roles between HHS and DHS were not fully implemented during this pandemic. Officials from both HHS and DHS told us that once it became clear that the H1N1 pandemic required primarily a public health response, HHS was responsible for most of the key activities.[44] Nevertheless, some state officials cited concerns about the shared federal leadership roles in the early days of the pandemic response. Specifically, officials we interviewed in four of the five states said that during that period, HHS and DHS did not effectively coordinate their release of information to their state contacts. As a result, state officials reported receiving large volumes of information—often through multiple daily conference calls or via e-mail—from both federal agencies. The amount of information—which was sometimes the same information and sometimes inconsistent—was overwhelming, according to these state officials. For example, representatives from the Georgia Emergency Management Agency told us that at one point DHS officials were telling states that confirmation of H1N1 influenza cases needed to be completed by a laboratory, which was the initial CDC guidance, while HHS officials were telling states they could confirm H1N1 cases by laboratories or an analysis of symptoms that the patient was experiencing, which was the revised CDC guidance at the end of August 2009. Officials in Vermont, Washington, and Georgia told us that over time it appeared to them that HHS—and primarily HHS's CDC—took the lead in communicating about H1N1 and, accordingly, the number of calls and information sources decreased.

Prior Federal Funding and Planning Built Capacity and Interagency Relationships, which Facilitated the Federal Response

Federal funding and planning for pandemic preparedness prior to the onset of the H1N1 pandemic paid off by building capacity in several areas, including (1) vaccine production, (2) influenza diagnosis, and (3) antiviral drug development and stockpiling. First, the retrofitted influenza vaccine manufacturing facilities that HHS funded doubled the production capacity for

H1N1 vaccine at two vaccine manufacturers, according to HHS.[45] These two manufacturers told us that the expanded capacity enabled them to start production of the H1N1 vaccine while they finished their production of seasonal influenza vaccine. Second, one of the influenza diagnostic tests that HHS's pandemic planning efforts helped fund detected the first case of H1N1 influenza as part of a clinical trial at the Naval Health Research Laboratory in San Diego, California. Third, the antiviral drug Peramivir— which was developed using pandemic preparedness funds—was made available for the first time during the H1N1 pandemic, and CDC delivered about 2,100 5-day treatment courses to hospitals.[46] Also, according to CDC officials involved in the response, no national shortage of adult antiviral drugs occurred during the H1N1 pandemic, which may have been due in part to prior federal and state stockpiling efforts. There was, however, a shortage of pediatric antiviral drugs in the fall of 2009.

Through interagency planning efforts, federal officials built relationships that helped facilitate the federal response to the H1N1 pandemic. Officials from HHS's ASPR and CDC, DHS, and Education stated that these interagency meetings, working together on existing pandemic and nonpandemic programs, and exercises conducted prior to the H1N1 pandemic built relationships that were valuable for the H1N1 pandemic response. Specifically, HHS officials said that federal coordination during the H1N1 pandemic was much easier because of these formal networks and informal relationships built during pandemic planning activities and exercises. For example, in developing the national pandemic strategy and national pandemic implementation plan, the HSC convened regular interagency meetings to facilitate cooperation and coordination across the federal government to prepare for an influenza pandemic. The NSS continued to hold these interagency meetings during the H1N1 pandemic response. Also, Education and CDC officials told us that in addition to these formal meetings, they had existing working relationships with each other that had been built while developing and managing a range of programs. Finally, officials from HHS, DHS, and other agencies held joint pandemic exercises to test various parts of the plan. As we have previously reported, DHS officials have said that exercises offer the best opportunity—short of actual emergencies—to determine if plans are understood and work.[47] DHS officials stated that as a result of pandemic planning and exercises, DHS and other federal agency officials knew whom to contact within federal agencies when H1N1 influenza emerged. NSS and HHS officials reported to us in April 2011 that many of the same departments and officials are meeting regularly as part of a new group to discuss emerging pandemic threats.

Planning efforts also allowed federal and state officials to build upon preexisting relationships that were useful during the pandemic response. These relationships had been built through daily interactions implementing grant programs, developing state and local pandemic plans, and working together in pandemic planning exercises. For example, CDC held a pandemic planning exercise with other federal officials and 11 state and local jurisdictions in October 2008. During this exercise, officials practiced responding to a pandemic influenza situation. A senior CDC official said that preexisting relationships with states and localities allowed them to be frank, informal, and comfortable with each other when responding to the H1N1 pandemic. Georgia health officials told us that they spoke to CDC project officers daily during the H1N1 response to provide real-time situational awareness because of their relationships formed prior to the pandemic. Washington health officials also said that existing relationships with CDC officials helped their response efforts. Specifically, CDC revised school closure guidance based in part on experiences with school closures in Seattle, Washington. This revised guidance recognized that because the disease severity of H1N1 influenza was similar to that of seasonal influenza and the virus had already spread within communities, the focus was on keeping sick children and staff at home rather than closing schools as a way to stop the spread of the virus.

Failure to Meet Public Expectations about Vaccine Availability Diminished Government Credibility, but Some Practices for H1N1 Vaccine Distribution Were Reported to Be Valuable

H1N1 Vaccine Was Not Widely Available when Expected nor when Demand Was Highest

By the time H1N1 vaccine was widely available, the peak of H1N1 influenza activity had passed and many individuals were no longer as interested in getting vaccinated.[48] (See fig. 3.) The national pandemic implementation plan established a goal of expanding influenza vaccine manufacturing surge capacity for the production of pandemic vaccines to allow for the entire domestic population to be able to receive a vaccine within 6 months of a pandemic declaration.[49]

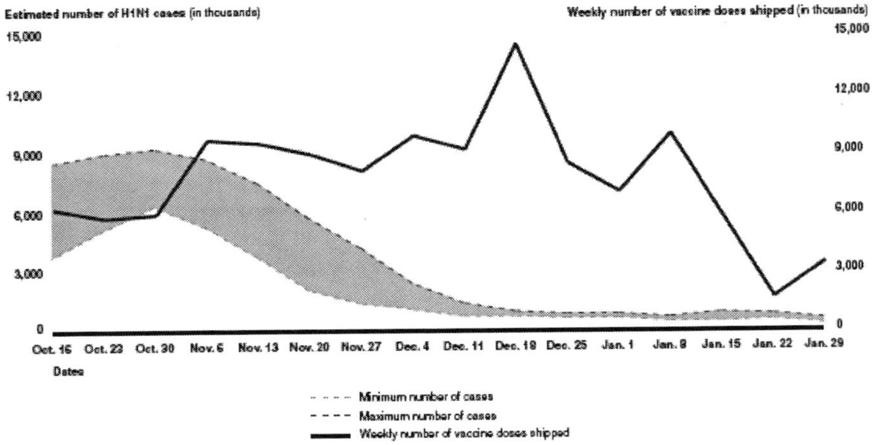

Source: GAO analysis of CDC data.

Figure 3. H1N1 Influenza Activity and Vaccine Availability, October 2009 through January 2010.

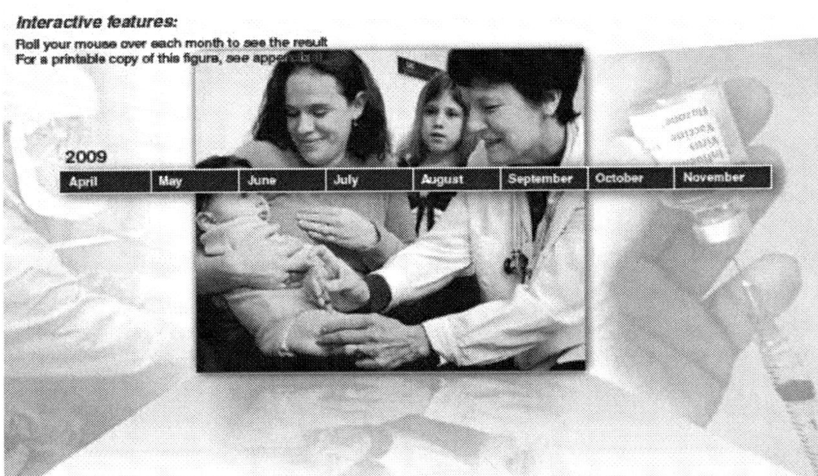

Sources: GAO analysis; James Gathany (photos).

Figure 4. Key Events Related to 2009 H1N1 Vaccine Production and Distribution in the United States, April 2009 through November 2009.

During the H1N1 pandemic, the H1N1 vaccine was first available in the United States in October 2009, or almost 4 months after WHO's pandemic declaration, but was not widely available for all who wanted to be vaccinated until late December 2009. (See fig. 4 for a timeline of key events related to H1N1 vaccine production and distribution.) A RAND Corporation study found that at the onset of influenza activity, about half of adults were willing to get vaccinated,[50] but after the vaccine became available, CDC reported that only about 23 percent of adults actually were vaccinated.[51]

The credibility of all levels of government was diminished when the amount of vaccine available to the public in October 2009 did not meet expectations set by federal officials. During the summer of 2009, HHS conveyed to state and local jurisdictions, and to the public, that a robust H1N1 vaccine supply, about 120 million to 160 million doses, was expected to be available in October 2009. Ultimately, only about 23 million doses of H1N1 vaccine were allocated for ordering by states and local jurisdictions at the end of October 2009, and because of the time required to order and ship the vaccine, fewer than 17 million doses were shipped out that month.[52] Consequently, the public had an unfavorable view of the federal government's ability to provide the country with the H1N1 vaccine. A Gallup survey of U.S. adults from early November 2009, found that 54 percent of adults said the federal government was doing a poor (41 percent) or very poor (13 percent) job of providing the country with adequate supplies of the vaccine.[53] An ASTHO report echoed that loss of government credibility also was a concern at the state level. ASTHO concluded that state health department officials felt that dealing with slow and variable vaccine delivery and shifting messages about vaccine availability overshadowed all of their other response activities.[54] For example, when vaccine availability was less than anticipated, state and local health departments had to cancel planned and publicized mass vaccination clinics and change their messages to the public about vaccination at a time when H1N1 influenza activity was peaking. Also, at the local level, health department officials in Fulton County, Georgia, stated that they canceled several school-based vaccination clinics because they lacked the H1N1 vaccine. According to these officials, once the H1N1 vaccine became available, parents were not interested in vaccinating their children because H1N1 influenza activity had already peaked in the area.

HHS has acknowledged that the H1N1 vaccine arrived too late in the response and noted the department is actively looking for ways to shorten the time required for vaccine production. The agency plans to use a portion of the remaining 2009 pandemic supplemental funds for these efforts. According to the Director of BARDA—who during the H1N1 pandemic response was responsible for overseeing the largest development and production of vaccine in U.S. history—once HHS staff were positioned at the vaccine manufacturing plants and manufacturers were required to report their time frames in a standard manner, HHS had a better understanding of the vaccine manufacturing process and the estimates for vaccine availability became more accurate in November 2009. A senior CDC official acknowledged that the uncertainty in the initial vaccine estimates was not adequately conveyed to state and local jurisdictions in the early days of the response effort.

State and Local Jurisdictions Valued Flexibility in Implementing Vaccination Campaigns, but Differences across Neighboring Jurisdictions Led to Public Confusion

Officials from state and local jurisdictions valued the flexibility that they had to implement their vaccine distribution plans. Although the federal government purchased the H1N1 vaccine and ACIP recommended that states and local jurisdictions initially provide it to individuals in the target groups, CDC allowed for state and local flexibility over vaccine distribution plans. NACCHO, as well as participants in a series of IOM workshops, reported that officials from state and local jurisdictions welcomed the flexibility to determine their own vaccine distribution plans. At the same time, state officials acknowledged that the flexibility, while appreciated, also led to confusion or the appearance of inequity, especially when the public became aware of different approaches taken in neighboring jurisdictions.[55] Participants in an IOM workshop reported that officials from jurisdictions that had approaches different from neighboring jurisdictions found it hard to communicate to the public about why one county or state was vaccinating a certain subset of their population while another was not.[56] For example, Snohomish County, Washington, initially included teachers in its target groups and conducted mass vaccination clinics, while neighboring Seattle-King County did not include teachers and distributed its initial supply of vaccine to physicians who were to vaccinate their patients. An official from the Seattle-King County health department reported that the public was confused by the differences. Washington health officials told us that they attempted to coordinate use of the target groups at the state level, but because local jurisdictions ultimately have control of local public health policies in the state, there were still differences between counties in implementation. Also, Vermont officials told us that the neighboring state of New York began vaccinating the general public beyond the target groups while Vermont was still waiting for guidance from CDC to widen its distribution.

CDC attempted to minimize confusion and anxiety by alerting the public that there would be differences in distribution methods. CDC's spokespeople emphasized this variation in the majority of the 18 press briefings that the agency held from September 2009 through December 2009 that we reviewed. A senior CDC official acknowledged the confusion resulting from allowing state and local flexibility, but noted that the agency would make the same decision again because of the importance of local public health decision making.

Use of a Central Vaccine Distributor Was Generally Cited as an Effective Practice, but Limitations in Sizes of Vaccine Orders Was Cited as Problematic

CDC used a central vaccine distributor—building off the existing Vaccines for Children program—and this practice was generally cited as effective by association and state officials.[57] The Vaccines for Children program's central distributor shipped the H1N1 vaccine from regional distribution centers that received the H1N1 vaccines from five vaccine manufacturers to individual providers or organizations identified by state and local jurisdictions. State and local health officials, in conjunction with professional associations such as the American Medical Association, identified providers who signed agreements to administer the H1N1 vaccine, including providers who had not previously participated in the Vaccines for Children program, such as obstetricians, gynecologists, and other physicians who treat and immunize adults. According to CDC officials, once H1N1 vaccine arrived at the central distributor's regional distribution centers, 95 percent of the ordered doses of H1N1 vaccine were shipped out in accordance with CDC's contract.[58] An official with the Association of Immunization Managers, which represents immunization program managers in state and local jurisdictions, involved in the response reported that use of the central distributor was a "best" practice during the H1N1 pandemic response because the central distributor was already in place and in operation. This official noted that she did not hear any issues or complaints from her association's members about the use of the central distributor. Officials from four of the states we contacted also noted that the central distributor worked well. Alternatively, CDC could have shipped the H1N1 vaccine out to SNS receiving sites in states; CDC's prior pandemic planning had focused on direct distribution by manufacturers to a limited number of state health department–designated sites. However, officials had decided that using a private distributor—that routinely distributes seasonal influenza and other vaccines—was a preferable method. CDC officials stated that because of the success of the central distributor during the H1N1 pandemic, CDC now views this method as the most efficient and effective method of vaccine distribution. State officials in two states reported that using the SNS sites instead of the central distributor would have caused logistical challenges.

While the use of a central vaccine distributor was generally cited as an effective practice by state and local health officials during the H1N1 pandemic, some state health officials noted challenges with the distribution process. Specifically, some state officials said that the central distributor's 100-dose minimum shipment requirement caused problems. As part of its contract with CDC, the central distributor required that shipments to each site include a minimum of 100 doses of H1N1 vaccine. Officials in three of the five states we contacted, as well as the U.S. Virgin Islands, told us that the 100-dose minimum ordering requirement caused difficulties because they had to break down the 100-dose shipments into smaller shipments so they could be shipped to smaller vaccine providers. Texas officials told us that the state hired a third-party contractor to receive and repackage the shipments for smaller vaccine providers. ASTHO also cited this issue as a challenge, noting that the dosage order requirements caused delays in some providers receiving the H1N1 vaccine.[59] According to CDC officials, at the time that they were negotiating the distribution contract, the possibility existed that up to 600 million doses of H1N1 vaccine would need to be distributed as quickly and efficiently as possible, a magnitude that was unprecedented and untested.[60] At that time, CDC and the distributor determined that it would be inefficient and even cost prohibitive for the contractor to hire the additional staff to break packages into smaller units for distribution.

Public Surveys Generally Found CDC's Public Communication Campaign to Be Effective, but Communication Materials Were Not Accessible for All Populations

Public Surveys Found CDC's Communication Campaign to Be Effective

Public surveys, state officials, and representatives from professional associations generally found CDC's public communication campaign to be effective. To gauge the effectiveness of its communication campaign and other aspects of the H1N1 response, CDC and others contracted with the Harvard School of Public Health to conduct regular surveys of the public regarding the H1N1 response. One study, conducted as part of this initiative in March 2010 and April 2010 with a nationally representative sample of U.S. adults aged 18 years and older, found that 70 percent of adults rated CDC's H1N1 influenza communication campaign as excellent (25 percent) or good (45 percent).[61]

Ratings of the communication campaign did not differ considerably among different ethnic groups. Further, more than half of adults reported seeing or hearing the key H1N1 protection and prevention messages, which included messages suggesting that people should get the H1N1 vaccine, wash their hands or use hand sanitizer frequently, stay home from work or school if sick, and cough or sneeze into one's elbow or shoulder. A professional association official as well as state health officials from three of the states we contacted also credited these personal infection control messages when we asked them about CDC's communication with the public. The same survey found that 89 percent of adults said they would trust CDC a great deal (59 percent) or somewhat (30 percent) for information about protecting themselves or their families from H1N1 influenza.

According to CDC officials, the agency's communication with the public was based on the agency's decision to be transparent and open with the public about both known and unknown information. CDC's crisis communication principles—which it formally articulated in its H1N1 communication plan—emphasize transparency and acknowledgment of uncertainty, as well as a commitment to frequent updates as new information emerges.[62] Specifically, CDC established four goals during the pandemic to guide communication efforts:

- Provide timely, accurate, and credible information about the public health threat and government actions to prevent 2009 H1N1 influenza and mitigate its impact.
- Increase public awareness, knowledge, and adoption of influenza prevention, mitigation, and treatment recommendations. These recommendations included promotion of vaccines, community measures, personal and institutional infection control, and the correct use of antiviral drugs.
- Guide public expectations for change and variability related to prevention and mitigation recommendations.
- Protect the health of the public while minimizing social, economic, and educational disruption.

CDC held frequent press briefings to provide timely dissemination of new information on the evolving situation. For example, during the early days of the H1N1 outbreak, CDC held almost daily press briefings. Officials from all five states we contacted and the National Governors Association noted that the agency's spokespeople throughout the H1N1 pandemic were generally effective. The Director of the Center for Infectious Disease Research and Policy at the

University of Minnesota noted that CDC's communication campaign gave the public the sense that the federal government was in charge of the pandemic response. CDC also held a 2- day conference in August 2009 to educate the media about influenza and what the fall influenza season could entail. CDC officials said the conference provided context for the media representatives in attendance, fostered an environment of transparency, and established a relationship between media and CDC officials. In addition to the interactions with the media, CDC used a variety of tools to reach the public directly (see fig. 5). According to CDC officials, communications was an integrated part of the response, with senior communications officials from across the agency represented when all major decisions were made. These officials noted that the inclusion of these representatives when decisions were being made allowed for a two-way conversation where policy experts took into consideration the perceptions and concerns of the public.

CDC officials reported using a number of different tools to reach the public with their messages:

- CDC used traditional media outlets, such as newspapers, television, and radio.
- CDC used the flu.gov Web site to provide a single source of information about the H1N1 pandemic.
- CDC introduced content syndication, which allowed CDC to automatically update entities that subscribed to CDC and CDC's Web sites when CDC updated its own information.
- CDC used social media, such as Twitter and blogs, to share information.

Source: GAO analysis.

Figure 5. CDC Communication Tools Used during the H1N1 Pandemic Response.

In addition, state and local jurisdictions appreciated CDC's efforts to keep them informed of ongoing changes. For example, CDC had representatives from professional associations representing state and local health officials at its Emergency Operations Center during the second wave of the pandemic, which occurred in fall 2009.[63] This was the first time that this type of involvement had happened, according to the association and CDC officials. According to CDC officials, the inclusion of these organizations helped foster transparency and allowed for the federal government to better understand the perspectives of state and local jurisdictions. Officials from Texas's health department noted that CDC shared talking points with them before conference calls. These officials told us that this gave them credibility because they were aware of information before it was shared broadly. In addition, Georgia health officials told us that they appreciated the frequent information sharing from sources such as CDC phone calls with states and the Web site *flu.gov*, which disseminated information during the H1N1 pandemic.

State and Local Jurisdictions Cited Need for More Timely Communication Materials for Non-English-Speaking Populations

State and local jurisdiction officials we spoke with wanted CDC to provide more communication materials for non-English-speaking populations. Specifically, three of the states we contacted—as well as the National Indian Health Board—reported that in order to serve their populations, they needed CDC communication materials, including posters and public service announcements, translated into additional languages in a more timely manner. Some state officials and ASTHO also expressed that it would be more efficient for CDC to translate materials once than for each state or local jurisdiction to spend the resources to do so individually or to rely on nonexperts for translation. Officials in Seattle-King County, Washington, reported that they had to translate materials into 20 languages to meet their jurisdiction's needs. Similarly, in Vermont, health officials reported that they needed to translate and print materials into 7 languages, only 2 of which were included in CDC's translated materials. The Vermont health officials told us that the process of translation took several weeks, which they said affected the vaccination rates among these populations. Following the H1N1 pandemic, an ASTHO report recommended that the federal government routinely take the lead in translating pandemic materials into multiple languages.[64]

CDC officials explained the range of translation services they offered, but also noted that they could take additional measures to assist states with translation. CDC communications officials said that the agency translated its television and radio public service announcements about the H1N1 pandemic into Spanish and translated written materials into a range of languages.[65] CDC officials explained that they select the range of translation services they will offer from a list of over 100 languages and explained that these selections are based on the geography of the situation, input from state and local public information officers, input from stakeholders, and information from the searches that users complete on the CDC Web site. CDC officials also told us that because information about the pandemic was changing so quickly, it was challenging for CDC to translate all of the information in a timely manner. A CDC official noted that the agency could serve some additional roles in facilitating translation for states, such as working with state partners to establish a clearinghouse for already-translated materials as well as a plan to identify and address translation gaps that avoids duplication of effort and helps ensure consistency and accuracy. For translation into additional languages, CDC officials noted that states could use the PHER grant funds.

Deployment of the SNS Met the Established Goal, but Gaps in Planning Were Identified

SNS Deployment Met Goal, but State and Local Jurisdictions Cited Need for Improved Communication from CDC on the Timing and Content of Shipments

While deployment of supplies from the SNS met the established goal, officials from state and local jurisdictions reported a need for improved communication about the timing and contents of shipments. Five days after the initial diagnosis of H1N1 influenza, on April 26, 2009, CDC released a quarter of the antiviral drugs and other supplies—including 11 million courses of antiviral drugs and 39 million face masks and respirators, gowns, and gloves. Seven days later, on May 3, 2009, all states and local jurisdictions—except two of the Pacific Island territories—had received their SNS allocations.[66] Officials we interviewed in three states and participants in a series of IOM workshops noted that officials from state and local jurisdictions did not always know when SNS shipments would be arriving or what would be included in the shipments.[67] For example, Nebraska officials reported that they were told a shipment would be arriving at 6:30 a.m., but the materials arrived earlier—at 2:30 a.m. Nebraska officials were able to meet the delivery trucks with a team of staff, but the shipment contained only two cases of gloves, which was not what they anticipated. Officials from Texas reported that SNS delivery schedules were often not adhered to and the lists of what would be in the shipments were incorrect. Georgia officials reported that they were not informed before the SNS supplies arrived at state warehouses, which meant that they were not able to provide the planned security for the supplies.

CDC officials told us that they took a variety of steps during the second wave of the pandemic to improve collaboration with the states about the timing and contents of the SNS shipments. Specifically, they noted that they recognized that states were not operating on 24-hour schedules, as had been assumed in prior SNS planning efforts. Accordingly, CDC's SNS officials explained that they changed their delivery schedules to only deliver supplies during working hours. They also told us that when they contacted the states to coordinate the timing of SNS shipments, they also provided more information on the contents of the shipments. These officials also told us that they revised the SNS procedures to institutionalize these measures.

Not All Models of Respirators in the SNS Were Commonly Used, and Guidelines Were Conflicting

According to some state and local officials, one gap in SNS planning was that the respirators provided through the SNS were different from those used by state and local jurisdictions. IOM reported in its summary of a series of workshops that the respirator models—also called N95 respirators—that state and local jurisdictions (and subsequently hospitals and other health care facilities) received from the SNS were not the same as the models hospitals regularly used, nor was a standard model provided, which necessitated additional fit testing by recipients.[68] To be optimally effective, respirators require a tight facial seal, thus individual "fit testing" is required. In Washington, state officials and Snohomish County officials told us that they received an unfamiliar brand of respirators in their SNS shipment that required fit testing of equipment that they did not have available. ASTHO also reported that state and local officials found the SNS respirators problematic and reported that states did not know which models of respirators were in the SNS or which models would be delivered.[69] CDC officials responsible for the SNS acknowledged problems with familiarity with the models of respirators in the SNS and reported that they are looking into a range of solutions, including standardizing the type of respirators included in the SNS and providing a catalog of stored supplies to states.[70] An official from CDC's National Institute for Occupational Safety and Health told us that the institute is also researching the next generation of respirators for health care workers. Another CDC division is also working with partners to develop reusable masks specifically designed for health care settings.

State and local government officials were also confused by conflicting federal and nonfederal guidance on the need for health care workers to wear respirators. In 2007, HHS and the Department of Labor issued joint guidance recommending that health care workers use respirators when in close contact with patients who have confirmed or suspected influenza during a pandemic. In May 2009, CDC released infection control guidance for clinicians to use during the H1N1 outbreak that was consistent with the 2007 guidance. Further, a September 2009 study by IOM, which was requested by CDC and Department of Labor's OSHA, agreed with the existing 2007 guidance in the specific case of H1N1 influenza.[71] However, conflicting guidance by other groups caused confusion during the H1N1 pandemic. The Infectious Disease Society of America and WHO recommended that health care workers only be required to wear respirators during health care procedures that involve specific types of exposure, such as intubation,[72] resuscitation, or open suctioning of the respiratory tract. According to HHS officials, many clinicians preferred to adhere to the infection control procedures that they use for seasonal influenza. An ASTHO report noted that conflicts in guidance left health care and other affected organizations wondering which guidance to follow. Further, ASTHO reported that the requirement for health care workers to wear respirators resulted in supply shortages and required extra time and resources by health care facilities for fit testing.73 Officials from OSHA told us, and IOM reported, that the available guidance is contradictory because scientific research about routes of disease transmission and respirator efficacy is inconclusive. Additionally, OSHA officials acknowledged that there is currently an inadequate supply of respirators to meet demand if all health care workers followed the existing guidance.

SNS Planning Did Not Account for the Need for Long-Term Storage or Recovery of Unused SNS Materials

Another gap identified in SNS planning was related to long-term storage of unused SNS materials. During the response to the H1N1 pandemic, some of the state officials that we interviewed told us that they did not use all of their SNS supplies. Nebraska officials, for example, told us that they only used a few cases of SNS materials that they received and were storing the remaining SNS materials in a state facility. Vermont officials reported that they did not use all of their SNS supplies and, as a result, were paying for storage as of June 2010. These state officials told us that they did not know what to do with the remaining SNS items. A CDC official who works on SNS issues acknowledged that the federal government did not have plans for the handling of states' unused SNS materials. He said that long-term inventory management or return of SNS items to the federal government was not a part of SNS exercises because distribution plans were based on a more severe pandemic scenario or other emergencies where all available supplies would be used quickly after distribution. The CDC official said that the agency needs to plan for alternative scenarios when the commercial market may be able to handle the demand for items in the SNS.

In June 2010, HHS's FDA provided guidance to CDC on the disposal of materials in anticipation of the end of emergency use authorizations, which allowed potentially helpful countermeasures to be used for unapproved uses to protect the public health. For example, FDA advised that states could hold on to respirators for a possible future public health emergency or distribute the respirators to be used in a manner consistent with their clearances. In its guidance, FDA also advised that state officials could continue to hold onto FDA-specified antiviral drugs for use in a future emergency situation, provided that they are stored appropriately.

Federal Agencies Are Completing After-Action Reports; Next Steps, Including Sharing with Key Stakeholders, Are Unclear

Federal Agencies Were Asked to Complete H1N1 Pandemic After-Action Reports by the NSS

According to the NSS, all federal agencies were asked to complete after-action reports appropriate to their level of involvement in the H1N1 pandemic response. The NSS relayed to us in November 2010 that while it did not establish guidelines for these after-action reports, it was monitoring the status of the reports. HHS officials told us that NSS last requested that HHS report on the status of its H1N1 after-action reports and follow-up activities in September 2010.

The NSS stated in April 2011 that it had not determined whether it would synthesize the federal agency after-action reports into a single governmentwide after-action report or if it will make the after-action reports available to key stakeholders, such as state and local governments. Nevertheless, a DHS official commented that sharing lessons from the reports with stakeholders would foster a spirit of government transparency and might help build stakeholder trust.

Officials from HHS, DHS, and Education confirmed that they are completing their H1N1 pandemic after-action reports. The departments took different approaches to collecting information for these reports, and as of spring

2011, it was unclear whether the final reports will be made publicly available or shared with key stakeholders.

- HHS's process for completing its after-action report involved soliciting information from other federal and state agencies, as well as other response partners, such as health care providers. The process included a survey of experts across the federal government who had knowledge of HHS's H1N1 pandemic response; in-depth interviews with experts to assess the agency's H1N1 pandemic response; and stakeholder engagement sessions, conducted via webinars, with entities such as states, localities, private sector partners, and national trade associations. According to HHS officials, as of April 2011, the HHS after-action report was being reviewed within the department. HHS officials also reported that the dissemination plans for the report were not finalized. HHS officials did report that the agency incorporated lessons learned from the H1N1 pandemic into its update of the National Vaccine Plan, which describes initiatives to enhance education on the safety of vaccines and vaccination practices and to assist providers and the public in making informed decisions regarding vaccination.[74] In addition to the department's activities to prepare an after-action report, individual agencies have also taken steps to incorporate lessons learned into their planning activities. For example, in March 2011, CDC held an exercise to incorporate lessons learned from the H1N1 pandemic into planning for a possible future pandemic. During this exercise, CDC officials worked with representatives from other parts of HHS, associations, as well as states and local jurisdictions to simulate a response to an avian influenza pandemic, which would likely have a higher fatality rate than the H1N1 pandemic. FDA also revised its Emergency Operations Plan to reflect lessons from the agency's response to the pandemic. In addition, HHS officials told us that they plan to hold exercises with DHS to test shared leadership roles.
- DHS's after-action report process was led by the department's Office of Health Affairs. The Office of Health Affairs collected its information through a series of planning conferences, after-action discussions, and online surveys of agency officials.[75] The after-action report includes both strengths and areas for improvement to enhance future departmental performance during a pandemic or other all-hazards incident and is accompanied by a formal improvement plan. The DHS after action report was signed by the Secretary of Homeland Security on

May 20, 2011, and DHS officials told us that they have shared the report with the NSS. DHS officials also told us that they are in the process of developing their dissemination plans for the report's findings, including plans for sharing the findings with state and local governments.

- Education's after-action report will be based on information gathered during a working group meeting in February 2010 that included discussions of how Education responded to the H1N1 pandemic, what lessons were learned, and what the agency would do differently during another pandemic. As of March 2011, Education's after-action report had not been finalized, and Education did not have dissemination plans.
- OSHA officials also told us that they have completed an H1N1 after-action report.

NSS Reported Plans for a Broad Approach to Preparedness

In April 2011, a senior NSS official reported that the NSS had no plans to update the national pandemic implementation plan to incorporate lessons learned from the H1N1 pandemic response; however, these lessons may be incorporated into departments' individual operational plans. Instead of updating the national pandemic implementation plan, NSS officials reported that they are coordinating a larger effort to transition national preparedness from a dependence on fixed plans for specific threats to an approach based on the capabilities needed for a variety of hazards, or an all-hazards approach.[76] Furthermore, the NSS did not indicate how the after-action reports—and the associated lessons learned—will be used in future planning and preparedness efforts. Specifically, as discussed above, the NSS has not yet determined if it will share the lessons from the after-action reports with key stakeholders, such as state and local governments. As we have previously reported, stakeholder involvement during the planning process is important to ensure that both the federal government's and key stakeholders' responsibilities and resource requirements are clearly understood and agreed upon.[77] We have previously recommended that the HSC, which is supported by the NSS, update the national pandemic implementation plan to incorporate information from exercises and other experiences, such as the H1N1 pandemic.[78] Indeed, the National Response Framework—which outlines the manner in which the federal government responds to domestic incidents—specifies that evaluation and continual process improvement are cornerstones of effective preparedness.[79] It notes that improvement planning should develop specific recommendations for changes in practice, timelines for implementation, and assignments for completion.[80] In addition, DHS has defined the national preparedness system as a continuous cycle that involves four main elements: (1) policy and doctrine, (2) planning and resource allocation, (3) training and exercises, and (4) an assessment of capabilities and reporting.[81]

CONCLUSIONS

The H1N1 pandemic was the first human influenza pandemic in more than four decades. As such, it provided the first real-life opportunity to test and implement key aspects of the federal government's plans to respond to a pandemic, including those in the 2005 national pandemic strategy and the 2006 national pandemic implementation plan. Thus, it is important to capture the lessons from the experiences of this event, both in terms of response actions that worked as well as those that could be improved.

It is also imperative to learn from these lessons by incorporating them into future planning and exercising efforts so that the nation can be better prepared when the next influenza pandemic occurs. These lessons may also be more broadly applicable to other hazards or emergencies that require response measures, such as activation of the SNS. They are also relevant to key stakeholders, such as state governments, which were instrumental in this response and would play a key role in a future response. All sectors of society, including governments, nonprofit organizations, and the private sector, will need to be involved in preparedness for a future pandemic. Accordingly, key stakeholders will need to adjust their own plans and understand their critical roles in order to be prepared to work effectively under difficult and challenging circumstances.

These lessons also have some important limitations. Specifically, while the H1N1 pandemic provided the opportunity to test and implement many aspects of the federal government's plans to respond to a pandemic, not all parts of these plans—such as those dealing with critical infrastructure protection and implementing border and trade measures—were tested. In addition, the shared leadership structure was not fully tested, and states raised concerns about their brief experience with these shared leadership roles. HHS's and DHS's plans to test this structure will be an important step to addressing this gap. These aspects may prove to be necessary in response to a future pandemic, given that avian and other strains of influenza remain a threat.

Our review of the federal government's response to the H1N1 pandemic highlighted several key lessons:

- Planning and preparedness pay off. While the actual H1N1 outbreak and pandemic differed from the avian influenza pandemic scenario that was the basis for the planning, many of the funding and planning activities—including funding for vaccine production capacity, planning exercises, and interagency meetings prior to the H1N1 pandemic— positioned the government to respond effectively. The interagency working group, convened by the NSS, fostered relationships that proved advantageous during the response.
- Effective communication on the availability of vaccine is central to a successful response. Although the federal government was able to purchase and distribute millions of doses of H1N1 vaccine, the vaccine was not widely available when the public expected it and at the peak of demand. Because the failure to effectively manage public expectations can undermine government credibility, it is essential that vaccine production efforts be paired with effective communication strategies regarding the availability of the vaccine.
- Timely, accessible information from CDC is valuable. The public proved to be highly receptive to the information CDC disseminated regarding the pandemic and what individuals could do to reduce their susceptibility to H1N1 influenza. However, the effectiveness of communication materials was diminished for some non-English-speaking populations when translated materials were not available to them in a timely manner. We heard from state and local health jurisdictions that they need materials in more languages, and they suggested that communications would be more accurate and translated more efficiently if key materials were translated centrally.
- Given the key role of the SNS in a public health emergency, consideration of logistics, inventory, and different scenarios is important in planning for SNS deployment. The largest deployment of the SNS to date occurred during the H1N1 pandemic response, but several issues emerged because scenarios arose that had not been anticipated. Resolving these issues now—in planning for future SNS deployment—will allow for better use of SNS resources during the next public health emergency.

Novel strains of influenza, including avian influenza strains, will continue to pose the threat of an influenza pandemic that could be more severe than the H1N1 pandemic. Accordingly, the failure to learn from the federal government's response to the H1N1 pandemic could be costly in terms of lives and resources, regardless of whether future planning is specific to a pandemic scenario or if it is incorporated into a broader "all-hazards" planning scenario. Although the NSS has requested that federal agencies prepare after-action reports, NSS officials have not decided how they will work with HHS and DHS to incorporate these lessons into any future planning, as called for by the *National Response Framework*, or how they will share these lessons with key stakeholders.

RECOMMENDATIONS FOR EXECUTIVE ACTION

We recommend that the Homeland Security Council direct the National Security Staff to take the following two actions:

- In order to help the federal government prepare for a future influenza pandemic, work with the Departments of Health and Human Services and Homeland Security—as well as other federal agencies and state and local jurisdictions, as applicable—to update planning and exercising by incorporating lessons learned from federal agencies' H1N1 after-action reports and the lessons we identified from the H1N1 pandemic. These lessons may include
- developing communication strategies for better managing public expectations about pandemic vaccine availability while working to reduce the length of time required to produce a pandemic vaccine;
- identifying state and local jurisdictions' need for materials for non-English-speaking populations and examining ways to facilitate the timely and efficient translation of key communication materials; and
- updating SNS plans by identifying tools for tracking SNS supplies, ensuring that the supplies in the SNS meet the needs of states and local jurisdictions, and accommodating previously unanticipated scenarios, such as the need for possible long-term storage or recovery of unused supplies.
- In order to help key stakeholders prepare for a future influenza pandemic or other public health emergencies, work with the Departments of Health and Human Services and Homeland Security—as well as other federal agencies, as applicable—to share the relevant findings of their after-action reports with key stakeholders, such as state and local governments.

AGENCY COMMENTS AND OUR EVALUATION

We provided a draft report for review and comment to the Associate General Counsel for the NSS, which works on behalf of the HSC, as well as the Secretaries of Health and Human Services, Homeland Security, Labor, and Education. The Secretary of Education did not provide any formal comments.

A legal advisor to the NSS did not provide written comments to be included in the final report, but agreed that the NSS would take the report and its recommendations under advisement.

In written comments, the HHS Assistant Secretary for Legislation responded that HHS generally agreed with our findings, and stated that its forthcoming after-action report will highlight several of the key themes that we address in our report. He also noted that HHS is already taking actions to address some of our findings, such as, reducing the time needed to make a pandemic influenza vaccine available and examining ways to make financial resources available during an emergency to states and local jurisdictions. He also provided technical comments, on behalf of HHS, which we incorporated as appropriate.

In written comments, the Director of the DHS GAO/Office of the Inspector General Liaison Office stated that DHS remains committed to working with the HSC, the NSS, HHS, and other relevant stakeholders to fulfill its shared leadership responsibility for pandemic influenza response. He also provided technical comments, on behalf of DHS, which we incorporated as appropriate.

On behalf of the Department of Labor, the Assistant Secretary for Occupational Safety and Health responded that OSHA provided an important contribution to the federal pandemic response by protecting workers' safety and health during the H1N1 pandemic. The Assistant Secretary further explained that OSHA has drafted an after-action report, which explains that the full range of OSHA's training, education, enforcement, and public outreach programs were used to help employers and workers protect themselves at work during the H1N1 pandemic.

HHS, DHS, and OSHA's comments are reprinted in appendices III through V.

We are sending copies of this report to the HSC, the Secretary of Health and Human Services, the Secretary of Homeland Security, the Secretary of Education, the Secretary of Labor, and appropriate congressional committees. The report also is available at no charge on the GAO Web site at http://www.gao.gov.

If you or your staff have any questions about this report, please contact Bernice Steinhardt at (202) 512-6543 or steinhardtb@gao.gov or Marcia Crosse at (202) 512-7114 or crossem@gao.gov. Contact points for our Offices of Congressional Relations and Public Affairs may be found on the last page of this report. GAO staff who made major contributions to this report are listed in appendix VI.

Bernice Steinhardt
Director, Strategic Issues

Marcia Crosse
Director, Health Care

APPENDIX I: INFORMATION ON SELECTION CRITERIA FOR FIVE SELECTED STATES

To examine how states and local jurisdictions used the grant funds and interacted with federal departments during the response, we interviewed officials involved in the H1N1 pandemic response in a sample of five states: Georgia, Nebraska, Texas, Vermont, and Washington. We chose these states to provide insight into the experiences of a range of states; however, their experiences are not generalizable to all 50 states.

The sample of five states was selected to reflect a range of six characteristics:

- Interim vaccination rate for initial target groups
- Census region
- First week of reported widespread influenza activity
- Public Health Emergency Response (PHER) grant funding
- The 2008 population (in thousands)
- Public health structure

Table 3 lists data for each state on each characteristic.

Table 3. Data for Selected States

State	Interim vaccination rate for initial target groups (percentage)[a]	Census region	First week of reported widespread influenza activity[b]	PHER grant funding[c]	2008 Population (in thousands)[d]	Public health structure[e]
Georgia	22.7	South	5/09/2009	$39,253,852	9,686	Hybrid
Nebraska	39.6	Midwest	7/11/2009	$10,251,928	1,783	Hybrid
Texas	20.8	South	5/09/2009	$93,258,556	24,327	Hybrid
Vermont	52.5	Northeast	10/17/2009	$5,882,237	621	Centralized
Washington	37.5	West	9/19/2009	$27,920,746	6,549	Decentralized

Source: GAO analysis of Department of Health and Human Services, Association of State and Territorial Health Officials, and U.S. Census Bureau data.

[a] interim vaccination rate for initial target groups is based on reported vaccination rates from October 2009 through January 2010. See Centers for Disease Control and Prevention, "Interim Results: Influenza A (H1N1) 2009 Monovalent Vaccination Coverage – United States, October through January 2010," Morbidity and Mortality Weekly Report, vol. 59, no. 12 (April 2010), 363.

[b]This is the first week that the state reported widespread influenza activity based on CDC's FluView from April 11, 2009, through December 26, 2009.

[c]This shows the total PHER grant funding for PHER phases one through three, as reported in CDC guidance to states.

[d]This is based on data reported by the U.S. Census Bureau in the Statistical Abstract of the United States, 2008.

[e]This is based on the Association of State and Territorial Health Officials' Profile of State Public Health, Volume 1. In a centralized structure, state health departments provide local public health services. In a decentralized structure, local health departments often collaborate with, but are organizationally independent of, state public health departments. In a hybrid structure, consumers may receive public health services from either the state or through agencies organized or operated by local governments, depending on the jurisdiction. In some cases, in hybrid structures state and local health departments share responsibility for providing services at the local level.

APPENDIX II: FULL TEXT FOR FIGURES 1, 2, AND 4 ON LESSONS FROM THE H1N1 PANDEMIC

The following information appears as interactive content in the body of the report when viewed electronically.

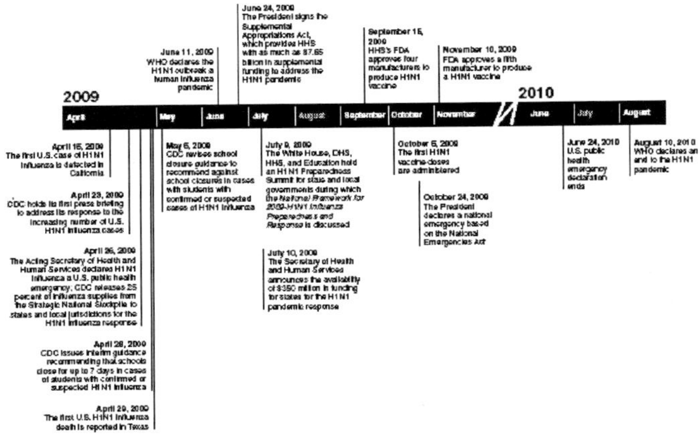

Source: GAO analysis.

Figure 6. Key Events Related to the H1N1 Pandemic in the United States, April 2009 through August 2010 (Printable Version).

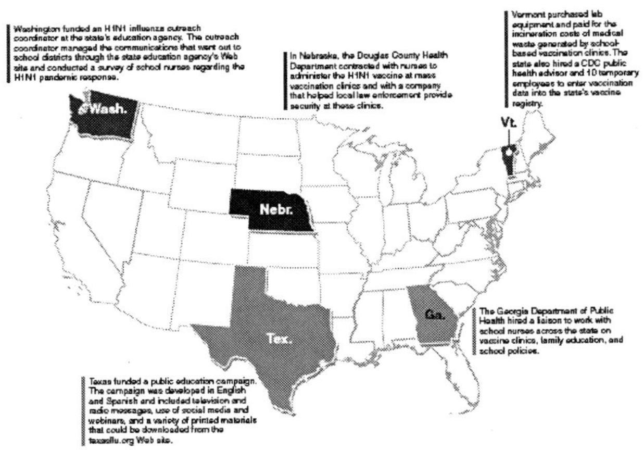

Sources: GAO analysis of state data; Map Resources (map).

Figure 7. Examples of Ways That State and Local Jurisdictions Used the PHER Grants (Printable Version).

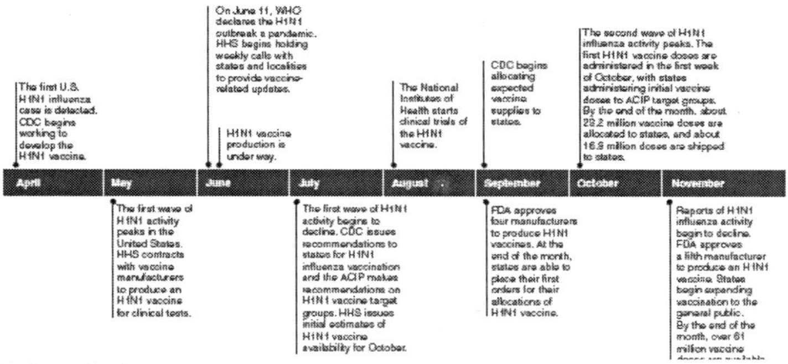

Source: GAO analysis.

Figure 8. Key Events Related to 2009 H1N1 Vaccine Production and Distribution in the United States, April 2009 through November 2009 (Printable Version).

APPENDIX III: COMMENTS FROM THE DEPARTMENT OF HEALTH AND HUMAN SERVICES

DEPARTMENT OF HEALTH & HUMAN SERVICES

Office of the Assistant Secretary for Legislation

Washington, D.C. 20201

JUN 01 2011

Bernice Steinhardt
Director, Strategic Issues
Marcia Crosse
Director, Health Care
U.S. Government Accountability Office
441 G Street N.W.
Washington, DC 20548

Dear Ms. Steinhardt and Ms. Crosse:

Attached are comments on the U.S. Government Accountability Office's (GAO) draft report entitled, "INFLUENZA PANDEMIC: Lessons From H1N1 Pandemic Should Be Incorporated into Future Planning" (GAO-11-632).

The Department appreciates the opportunity to review this report before its publication.

Sincerely,

Jim R. Esquea
Assistant Secretary for Legislation

Attachment

GENERAL COMMENTS OF THE DEPARTMENT OF HEALTH AND HUMAN SERVICES (HHS) ON THE GOVERNMENT ACCOUNTABILITY OFFICE'S (GAO) DRAFT REPORT ENTITLED, "INFLUENZA PANDEMIC: LESSONS LEARNED FROM H1N1 SHOULD BE INCORPORATED INTO FUTURE PLANNING" (GAO-11-632)

The Department appreciates the opportunity to review and comment on this draft report. We generally concur with the report and support the lessons highlighted in the report.

The forthcoming HHS Retrospective will in fact highlight several of these key themes: the value of planning and preparedness, the necessity of effective communication for a successful response, the importance of timely and accessible information, and deployment planning of the Strategic National Stockpile. Pandemic planning efforts going forward address these and other issues.

Below are a few examples of efforts currently underway to make systems improvements that will aid in pandemic response and the way the Department works with partners and improves capabilities for all threats:

- HHS is leading efforts to align preparedness grants across the Federal government, including the Hospital Preparedness Program (HPP) and Public Health Emergency Preparedness (PHEP) programs, to ensure more consistent administrative requirements. This will have the dual effect of making the process less burdensome to states and grantees and providing a unified Federal message on preparedness.

- The August 2010 Medical Countermeasures Review describes a plan for developing a nimble, flexible capability to produce not only pandemic vaccine but medical countermeasures (MCMs) for any threat. These recommendations are currently being implemented. The Biomedical Advanced Research and Development Authority (BARDA), the Centers for Disease Control and Prevention (CDC), the Food and Drug Administration (FDA), National Institute of Allergy and Infectious Diseases (NIAID) and vaccine industry partners are working together to address manufacturing and product release requirements that will speed availability of vaccines for distribution by up to 4-6 weeks. Also, BARDA awarded two more contracts supporting advanced development of recombinant influenza vaccines towards US licensure. Each of these contracts stipulate US-based manufacturing with the first dose of pandemic influenza vaccine available by 12 weeks post-onset and 50 million doses within 4 months.

- The 2010 President's Council of Advisers on Science and Technology's "Report to the President on Reengineering the Influenza Vaccine Production Enterprise to Meet the Challenges of Pandemic Influenza" made recommendations on ways to speed the availability of influenza vaccine during a pandemic. The Public Health Emergency Medical Countermeasures Enterprise (PHEMCE) has acted on many of these recommendations. For example, BARDA has issued advanced research and development contracts to several manufacturers developing next-generation recombinant influenza vaccines that may shorten development times considerably, and BARDA, CDC, and the National Institutes of Health (NIH) are working together and with industry to optimize vaccine seed strain production and develop faster approaches to required sterility and

GENERAL COMMENTS OF THE DEPARTMENT OF HEALTH AND HUMAN SERVICES (HHS) ON THE GOVERNMENT ACCOUNTABILITY OFFICE'S (GAO) DRAFT REPORT ENTITLED, "INFLUENZA PANDEMIC: LESSONS LEARNED FROM H1N1 SHOULD BE INCORPORATED INTO FUTURE PLANNING" (GAO-11-632)

potency testing that together could speed availability of vaccines for distribution by up to 4-6 weeks.

- Learning from the challenges related to pandemic vaccine availability estimates early in the 2009 H1N1 response, efforts are underway to improve situational awareness of vaccine production for future events. As mentioned in the report, increased coordination between HHS staff and vaccine manufacturers in November 2009 resulted in improved vaccine availability estimates. HHS is incorporating the need for better communication and coordination into several areas: our planning efforts; between federal officials and vaccine manufacturers to ensure real-time situational awareness for vaccine production and availability; and between federal agencies, states, and local health departments to adequately convey uncertainties in initial vaccine estimates.

Based on experiences from the 2009 H1N1 pandemic and other recent emergencies, such as the Deepwater Horizon Oil Spill and the Haiti Earthquake, the Department recognizes the need to examine and potentially refine how financial resources are made available during an emergency event, and is currently identifying relevant barriers and challenges. Once complete, this analysis should identify additional administrative flexibilities for using federal funds during future emergencies. Additionally, recipients of the Public Health Emergency Preparedness Cooperative Agreement have also been asked to examine their jurisdiction's administrative processes and approaches to receive and use emergency funds to respond to emergency situations in a timely manner, identify relevant barriers, and planned actions to address those challenges.

Appendix IV: Comments from the Department of Homeland Security

U.S. Department of Homeland Security
Washington, DC 20528

Homeland Security

May 31, 2011

Bernice Steinhardt
Director, Strategic Issues
and
Marcia Crosse
Director, Health Care
U.S. Government Accountability Office
441 G Street, NW
Washington, DC 20548

Re: Draft Report, GAO-11-632, "INFLUENZA PANDEMIC: Lessons from H1N1 Pandemic Should be Incorporated Into Future Planning"

Dear Ms. Steinhardt and Ms. Crosse:

Thank you for the opportunity to review and comment on this draft report. The U.S. Department of Homeland Security (DHS) appreciates the U.S. Government Accountability Office's work in planning and conducting its review and issuing this report. The Department is pleased to note the report's positive acknowledgment that through interagency planning efforts, federal officials, including DHS, have built relationships that helped facilitate the federal response to the H1N1 pandemic—the first human influenza pandemic in more than four decades.

Although the report does not contain any recommendations specifically directed at DHS, the The Department remains committed to continuing to work with the Homeland Security Council, National Security Staff, the Department of Health and Human Services, and other relevant stakeholders to fulfill its shared federal leadership responsibility for pandemic influenza response.

Again, thank you for the opportunity to review and comment on this draft report. Technical comments are being provided under separate cover. We look forward to working with you on future Homeland Security issues.

Sincerely,

Jim H. Crumpacker
Director
Departmental GAO/OIG Liaison Office

APPENDIX V: COMMENTS FROM THE DEPARTMENT OF LABOR

U.S. Department of Labor

Assistant Secretary for
Occupational Safety and Health
Washington, D.C. 20210

JUN - 6 2011

Ms. Bernice Steinhardt, Director
Strategic Issues
Ms. Marcia Crosse, Director
Health Care
U.S. Government Accountability Office
441 G Street, N.W.
Washington, D.C. 20548

Dear Ms. Steinhardt and Ms. Crosse:

Thank you for the opportunity to comment on the Government Accountability Office's (GAO) proposed report, *Influenza Pandemic: Lessons from H1N1 Pandemic Should be Incorporated Into Future Planning*. The Occupational Safety and Health Administration (OSHA) would like to make a few points we believe are important and deserve more attention in the report.

On page 6 of the report, it states that in preparing this report, GAO reviewed documents and interviewed officials from OSHA "regarding guidance on the use of personal protective equipment". This short phrase minimizes OSHA's contribution to the federal pandemic response. In addition to the "guidance on the use of personal protective equipment", GAO could at least add "and the protection of workers' safety and health." OSHA served on the 2009 NSS-created 2009 H1N1 Flu Sub-Interagency Policy Committee and OSHA's draft After-Action Report states that "the full range of OSHA's training, education, enforcement and public outreach programs were used to help employers and workers protect themselves at work during this pandemic."

OSHA appreciates the opportunity to review and respond to GAO's draft report.

Sincerely,

David Michaels, PhD, MPH

APPENDIX VI. ACKNOWLEDGMENTS

In addition to the contacts named above, Sarah Veale, Assistant Director; Kim Yamane, Assistant Director; Lori Achman; Mallory Barg Bulman; George Bogart; Helen Desaulniers; Karin Fangman; David Fox; Cathleen Hamann; Seta Hovagimian; and Susan Sato made key contributions to this report.

End Notes

[1] As part of its overall mission to protect public health, this international entity monitors global influenza outbreaks and declares pandemics based on the pattern of outbreaks in its regions.

[2] Influenza pandemics occur when a new influenza virus emerges and spreads around the world, and most people do not have immunity. This definition is based on spread of the disease, not severity. Three pandemics occurred in the 20th century: the "Spanish flu" of 1918, which caused 500,000 deaths in the United States; the "Asian flu" of 1957, which caused 70,000 deaths in the United States; and the "Hong Kong flu" of 1968, which caused 34,000 deaths in the United States.

[3] Throughout this report, we use "H1N1 influenza" to refer to the 2009 H1N1 influenza. We also use "H1N1 pandemic" to refer to the 2009 H1N1 influenza pandemic.

[4] See Centers for Disease Control and Prevention, "Updated CDC Estimates of 2009 H1N1 Influenza Cases, Hospitalizations, and Deaths in the United States, April 2009 – April 10, 2010," http://www.flu.gov/individualfamily/about/h1n1/estimates_2009_h1n1.html (accessed Dec. 7, 2010).

[5] The HSC was established pursuant to Executive Order 13228, on October 8, 2001, for purposes of advising and assisting the President with respect to all aspects of homeland security and serving as a mechanism for ensuring (1) coordination of homeland security–related activities of executive departments and agencies and (2) effective development and implementation of homeland security policies. The Congress subsequently established the HSC for the purpose of more effectively coordinating the policies and functions of the federal government relating to homeland security. See Homeland Security Act of 2002, Pub. L. No. 107-296 (Nov. 25, 2002), 6 U.S.C. § 491 and § 494.

[6] Medical countermeasures are medications, biological products, or devices that treat, identify, or prevent harm from a biological or other agent that may cause a public health emergency. Medical countermeasures for use during an influenza pandemic may include vaccines, antiviral drugs, personal respirators, and influenza diagnostic tests. Vaccine, considered the first line of defense against influenza, is used to stimulate the production of an immune system response to protect the body from disease. Antiviral drugs are medications that can prevent or reduce the severity of a viral infection, such as influenza.

[7] On May 26, 2009, the President established the NSS, under the direction of the National Security Advisor, to integrate White House staff supporting national security and homeland security. The President stated that the NSS would support the HSC, and that the HSC would be maintained as the principal venue for interagency deliberations on issues that affect the security of the homeland, such as pandemic influenza. See *Statement by the President on the*

White House Organization for Homeland Security and Counterterrorism, http://www.whitehouse.gov/the_press_office/Statement-by-the-President-on-the-White-House-Organization-for-Homeland-Security-and-Counterterrorism(accessed May 9, 2011).

[8] Supplemental Appropriations Act, 2009, Pub. L. No. 111-32, 123 Stat. 1859, 1884-1886 (June 24, 2009). A supplemental appropriation is an act appropriating funds in addition to those already enacted in the annual appropriation act. Supplemental appropriations provide additional budget authority usually in cases where the need for funds is too urgent to be postponed until enactment of the regular appropriation bill.

[9] For this report, we use "states and local jurisdictions" to refer to state, local, and tribal governments, as well as territorial and insular areas. 10The SNS, managed by CDC, contains large quantities of medicine and medical supplies intended to protect and treat the public if there is a public health emergency that is severe enough that local supplies may be exhausted.

[11] Related products are listed at the end of this report.

[12] To measure spending, we reviewed the department's obligations. "Obligation" refers to a definite commitment by a federal agency that creates a legal liability to make payments immediately or in the future. Agencies incur obligations, for example, when they award grants or contracts.

[13] In states without a centralized public health structure, we also met with at least one local jurisdiction's health department.

[14] "Personal protective equipment" encompasses the specialized clothing and equipment worn by workers for protection against health and safety hazards. For health care personnel, personal protective equipment may include respirators, face masks, gloves, eye protection, face shields, gowns, and head and shoe coverings.

[15] The Center for Infectious Disease Research and Policy addresses public health preparedness and emerging infectious diseases response. The Association of Immunization Managers represents state, local, and territorial immunization program managers. The National Indian Health Board represents tribal governments—both those operating their own health care delivery systems through contracting and compacting and those receiving health care directly from the Indian Health Service.

[16] Department of Homeland Security, *National Response Framework* (Washington, D.C., January 2008), 32.

[17] The *National Strategy for Pandemic Influenza* (national pandemic strategy), released in 2005, provides a framework for planning efforts for how the country will prepare for, detect, and respond to an influenza pandemic. The strategy reflects the federal government's approach to the pandemic threat and is based on three pillars: (1) preparedness and communication, (2) surveillance and detection, and (3) response and containment. The *National Strategy for Pandemic Influenza Implementation Plan* (national pandemic implementation plan) published in 2006, further clarifies the roles and responsibilities of federal and nonfederal entities—including state, local, and tribal governments; the private sector; international partners; and individuals—to prepare themselves and their communities. The national pandemic implementation plan includes 324 action items to address the threat of a pandemic, most of which have been reported as completed.

[18] Pub. L. No. 109-148, 119 Stat. 2680, 2783, 2786 (Dec. 30, 2005), and Pub. L. No. 109-234, 120 Stat. 418, 479-80 (June 15, 2006).

[19] The federal stockpile of antiviral drugs includes oral formulations (Tamiflu), inhaler formulations (Relenza), and doses for pediatric patients.

[20] For a more detailed discussion of how the 2006 supplemental funds were spent for pandemic preparedness, see GAO, *Influenza Pandemic: Sustaining Focus on the Nation's Planning and Preparedness Efforts*, GAO-09-334 (Washington, D.C.: Feb. 26, 2009), 30.

[21] According to HHS officials, they received this document from the NSS in July 2009.

[22] Influenza pandemics can have successive waves of disease and last for up to 3 years.

[23] Specifically, FDA determined that a monovalent influenza vaccine, which protects against a single strain of influenza, manufactured according to the same process as licensed seasonal influenza vaccines—but formulated to contain the pandemic 2009 H1N1 influenza virus strain antigen—could be approved as a strain change supplement to existing licensed influenza vaccines. An antigen is the active substance in a vaccine that provides immunity by causing the body to produce protective antibodies to fight off a particular influenza strain. To be effective, an influenza vaccine must be created to match a specific influenza strain because influenza strains undergo minor genetic changes from year to year. The 2009 H1N1 influenza vaccine was separate from, and in addition to, the seasonal influenza vaccine for the 2009-2010 influenza season. In addition, manufacturers and the National Institutes of Health conducted clinical trials to determine the optimal dosage and number of doses that would be required to generate an immune response to 2009 H1N1 infection.

[24] Centers for Disease Control and Prevention, "Use of Influenza A (H1N1) 2009 Monovalent Vaccine: Recommendations of the Advisory Committee on Immunization Practices (ACIP)," *Morbidity and Mortality Weekly Report*, vol. 58, no. RR-10 (August 2009), http://www.cdc.gov/mmwr/preview/mmwrhtml/rr58e0821a1.htm (accessed Apr. 25, 2011). ACIP develops written recommendations for the routine administration of vaccines to children and adults in the civilian population. These recommendations include age for vaccine administration, number of doses and dosing interval, and precautions and contraindications.

[25] These recommendations, based on the epidemiology of H1N1 influenza and projected vaccine supply, were made to assist in planning and to alert providers and the public about who should be first to receive the vaccine. ACIP recommended the following five initial target groups: pregnant women, household contacts and caregivers for children younger than 6 months of age, health care and emergency services personnel, individuals from 6 months through age 24, and persons aged 25 through 64 with health conditions associated with higher risk of medical complications from influenza.

[26] The subset of the target groups included pregnant women, individuals living with or caring for children younger than 6 months of age, health care and emergency medical services personnel with direct patient contact, and children aged 6 months through 4 years or aged 5 through 18 years with chronic medical conditions.

[27] Centers for Disease Control and Prevention, "Final Estimates for 2009-10 Seasonal Influenza and Influenza A 2009 (H1N1) Monovalent Vaccination Coverage – United States, August 2009 through May 2010,"http://www.cdc.gov/flu/professionals/vaccination /coverage_0910estimates.htm (accessed Oct. 8, 2010).

[28] HHS reported that it transferred about $241.20 million to the Department of Defense, Department of Veterans Affairs, Department of State, and Department of Agriculture. Since HHS spent the majority of the 2009 supplemental appropriation, we did not determine how the $241 million transferred to these other departments was spent by them. We did not independently verify the amount of money that was transferred. The 2009 supplemental appropriation requires that all funds transferred to these other departments go toward purposes related to preparing for or responding to an influenza pandemic.

[29] Section 1826 of the Department of Defense and Full-Year Continuing Appropriations Act, 2011, rescinded $1.259 billion in contingent 2009 supplemental funds that the President had not yet designated to the Congress as emergency funds. Pub. L. No. 112-10, 125 Stat. 10, 162 (Apr. 15, 2011).

[30] To measure spending, we looked at the agency's obligations. "Obligation" refers to a definite commitment by a federal agency that creates a legal liability to make payments immediately or in the future. Agencies incur obligations, for example, when they award grants or contracts. Because payments are typically made as goods or services are received, the funds listed may not have been expended. Upon termination of a contract, unexpended funds may be deobligated and, depending on the terms of their appropriation, may remain available to the agency.

[31] Department of Health and Human Services, *Report to Congress: December 2010 Report, Pandemic Influenza Preparedness Spending* (Washington, D.C., February 2011). We did not independently verify information on obligations provided in the report.

[32] Adjuvants are substances that may be added to a vaccine to increase the body's immune response to the vaccine. While adjuvants were purchased by HHS as a precautionary measure, they were not used in the H1N1 vaccine.

[33] HHS purchased over 190 million doses of vaccine. Of these doses, over 156 million were made available for distribution to the U.S. public and the Department of Defense, 17 million were distributed internationally, and the remainder were not distributed.

[34] CDC awarded PHER grants to each of the 50 states; 4 local health departments (Chicago, Los Angeles County, New York City, and Washington, D.C.); and American Samoa, Guam, the Marshall Islands, Micronesia, Northern Mariana Islands, Palau, Puerto Rico, and the U.S. Virgin Islands. HHS also provided funds to hospitals, through states, as part of the Hospital Preparedness Program.

[35] Specifically, the first funding phase was for state and local jurisdictions to assess their capabilities for pandemic influenza response and to address gaps in vaccination, antiviral distribution and dispensing, community mitigation, laboratory, epidemiology, and surveillance activities. The second funding phase was for state and local jurisdictions to plan for the vaccination campaign. The third funding phase was for states to implement the mass vaccination campaign. The fourth and final funding phase was for targeting special, hard-to-reach populations for vaccination.

[36] Association of State and Territorial Health Officials, *Assessing Policy Barriers to Effective Public Health Response in the H1N1 Influenza Pandemic* (Arlington, Va., June 2010), 25.

[37] ASTHO, *Assessing Policy Barriers to Effective Public Health Response in the H1N1 Influenza Pandemic*, 25.

[38] National Association of County and City Health Officials, *H1N1 Policy Workshop Report* (Washington, D.C., June 2010), 5.

[39] Office of the Assistant Secretary for Preparedness and Response, *The Public Health Emergency Medical Countermeasures Enterprise Review: Transforming the Enterprise to Meet Long-Range National Needs* (Washington, D.C., August 2010), http://www.hhs.gov/nvpo/nvac /meetings/upcomingmeetings/korch_presentation.pdf (accessed June 21, 2011).

[40] Department of Health and Human Services, *Amended Spending Plan for 2009 Supplemental Funding*, as reported to the Congress in August 2010.

[41] GAO, *Influenza Pandemic: Monitoring and Assessing the Status of the National Pandemic Implementation Plan Needs Improvement*, GAO-10-73 (Washington, D.C.: Nov. 24, 2009).

[42] For more information, see GAO, *Influenza Pandemic: Opportunities Exist to Address Critical Infrastructure Protection Challenges That Require Federal and Private Sector Coordination*, GAO-08-36 (Washington, D.C.: Oct. 31, 2007).

[43] See GAO, *Influenza Pandemic: Further Efforts Are Needed to Ensure Clearer Federal Leadership Roles and an Effective National Strategy*, GAO-07-781 (Washington, D.C.: Aug. 14, 2007).

[44] At the onset of the H1N1 outbreak, the President's nominee for Secretary of Health and Human Services had not yet been confirmed. She was confirmed on April 28, 2009.

[45] Department of Health and Human Services, *Report to Congress: June 2010 Report, Pandemic Influenza Preparedness Spending* (Washington, D.C., June 2010).

[46] The antiviral drug Peramivir was made available under an emergency use authorization (EUA) during the H1N1 pandemic. Peramivir was the first investigational drug to be made available under an EUA. During the Peramivir EUA period, CDC reported that it received 1,371 requests for Peramivir and delivered a total of 2,129 5-day adult treatment courses from the SNS to 563 hospitals in the United States within 24 hours of receipt of request. A study found that Peramivir was associated with recovery in most patients hospitalized with severe pneumonia associated with H1N1 influenza. See J.E. Hernandez et al., "Clinical Experience in Adults and Children Treated with Intravenous Peramivir for 2009 Influenza A (H1N1) Under an Emergency IND Program in the United States," *Clinical Infectious Diseases*, vol. 52, no. 6 (2011), 695-706.

[47] GAO, *Disaster Response: Criteria for Developing and Validating Effective Response Plans*, GAO-10-969T (Washington, D.C.: Sept. 22, 2010).

[48] The geographic distribution of H1N1 influenza activity was most widespread during the weeks ending October 24, 2009, and October 31, 2009, when 48 of 50 states reported widespread influenza activity. Centers for Disease Control and Prevention, "Update: Influenza Activity – United States, 2009-10 Season," *Morbidity and Mortality Weekly Report*, vol. 59, no. 29, (2010).

[49] See Homeland Security Council, *National Strategy for Pandemic Influenza Implementation Plan,* (Washington, D.C., May 2006).

[50] J. Maurer, K.M. Harris, et al., "Does Receipt of Seasonal Influenza Vaccine Predict Intention to Receive Novel H1N1 Vaccine: Evidence from a Nationally Representative Survey of U.S. Adults," *Vaccine*, vol. 27 (2009), 5732-5734.

[51] Centers for Disease Control and Prevention, "Final Estimates for 2009-10 Seasonal Influenza and Influenza A 2009 (H1N1) Monovalent Vaccination Coverage – United States, August 2009 through May 2010," http://www.cdc.gov/flu/professionals/vaccination /coverage_0910estimates.htm (accessed Oct. 8, 2010).

[52] As of December 2010, HHS allocated 138 million doses to states and local jurisdictions, provided 2.7 million doses to the Department of Defense, and donated 16 million doses internationally. About 127 million doses were distributed to states and local jurisdictions, 11 million less than the amount allocated. Not all distributed vaccines were administered. 53Gallup, *In U.S., 20% of Parents Unable to Get H1N1 Vaccine for Child* (Nov. 10, 2009), http://www.gallup.com/poll/124220/Parents-Unable-H1N1-Vaccine-Child.aspx (accessed Apr. 26, 2011).

[54] ASTHO, *Assessing Policy Barriers to Effective Public Health Response in the H1N1 Influenza Pandemic*, 20.

[55] NACCHO, *H1N1 Policy Workshop Report*, 11.

[56] Institute of Medicine, *The 2009 Influenza Vaccination Campaign: A Summary of a Workshop Series* (Washington, D.C.: The National Academies Press, October 2010), 31. 57 Vaccines for Children is a federally funded program that provides vaccines at no cost to children who might not otherwise be vaccinated because of their families' inability to pay. The program, administered by CDC, distributes pediatric vaccines to states and health care providers.

[58] According to CDC officials, CDC's contract with the distributor specified that all doses of H1N1 vaccine needed to be shipped out on the day the order was placed.

[59] ASTHO, *Assessing Policy Barriers to Effective Public Health Response in the H1N1 Influenza Pandemic*, 17.

[60] Because initial information suggested that two doses of H1N1 vaccine might be required, initial estimates for the number of H1N1 doses that would need to be shipped included the possibility of up to 600 million doses.

[61] R. Blendon, G. SteelFisher, M. Bekheit, and M. Herrmann, "The Public's Response to H1N1: A Multiethnic Perspective," Harvard Opinion Research Program, Harvard School of Public Health, http://www.hsph.harvard.edu/research/horp/project-on-the-public-response-to-h1n1/(accessed Jan. 6, 2011).

[62] CDC developed an internal H1N1 communications plan to guide its communications efforts during the response.

[63] CDC's Emergency Operations Center is the agency's command center for monitoring and coordinating CDC's emergency response to public health threats in the United States and abroad.

[64] ASTHO, *Assessing Policy Barriers to Effective Public Health Response in the H1N1 Influenza Pandemic*, 28.

[65] According to CDC officials, CDC's guidance is typically translated into 5 languages—Spanish, Vietnamese, Chinese, French, and Tagalog—but that during the H1N1 pandemic, documents were also translated regularly into the following 12 languages determined in consultation with HHS's Office of Minority Health: Arabic, Russian, Japanese, Korean, German, Burmese, Italian, Somali, Khmer, Kirundi, Amharic, and Oromo.

[66] According to CDC's SNS officials, this time frame met CDC's established goal for timely release of the SNS supplies.

[67] Institute of Medicine, *Medical Countermeasures Dispensing: Emergency Use Authorizations and the Postal Model: Workshop Summary* (Washington, D.C.: The National Academies Press, October 2010), 16.

[68] IOM, *Medical Countermeasures Dispensing: Emergency Use Authorizations and the Postal Model: Workshop Summary,* 14.

[69] ASTHO, *Assessing Policy Barriers to Effective Public Health Response in the H1N1 Influenza Pandemic*, 23.

[70] CDC officials explained that the SNS respiratory devices they had purchased for the SNS were based on perceived urgency to rapidly acquire and store the first available N95 respirators and surgical masks using earlier pandemic preparedness funds. They acquired N95 respirators and surgical masks based on product availability and were not able to plan to procure specific models to match local hospital needs. During the H1N1 pandemic, the SNS shipped these N95 respirators and surgical masks to augment state and local capabilities.

[71] See Institute of Medicine, *Respiratory Protection for Healthcare Workers in the Workplace Against Novel H1N1 Influenza A: A Letter Report* (Washington, D.C.: The National Academies Press, Sept. 1, 2009), 4.

[72] Generally, intubation is the introduction of a tube into an individual's airway to facilitate breathing.

[73] ASTHO, *Assessing Policy Barriers to Effective Public Health Response in the H1N1 Influenza Pandemic*, 23.

[74] The *National Vaccine Plan* focuses on all vaccines, not solely influenza vaccines.

[75] In May 2009, the Secretary of Homeland Security submitted a memorandum to the White House with lessons learned from the first wave of the H1N1 pandemic and next steps to undertake in preparation for the expected second wave in the fall of 2009.

[76] The White House released Presidential Policy Directive 8 on March 30, 2011. This directive aims to facilitate an integrated, all-of-nation, capabilities-based approach to preparedness.

[77] GAO-07-781.

[78] GAO-07-781 and GAO-10-73.

[79] Issued by DHS in January 2008, the *National Response Framework* is the doctrine that guides how federal, state, local, and tribal governments, along with nongovernmental and private sector entities, will collectively respond to and recover from all hazards, including catastrophic disasters such as Hurricane Katrina.

[80] DHS, *National Response Framework*, 32.

[81] Department of Homeland Security, *National Preparedness Guidelines* (Washington, D.C., September 2007).

In: Influenza
Editor: Richard A. Colon
ISBN: 978-1-62100-174-4

Chapter 2

INFLUENZA VACCINE: FEDERAL INVESTMENTS IN ALTERNATIVE TECHNOLOGIES AND CHALLENGES TO DEVELOPMENT AND LICENSURE*

United States Government Accountability Office

WHY GAO DID THIS STUDY

Production delays for the 2009 H1N1 pandemic vaccine using the current egg-based production technology heightened interest in alternative technologies that could expand the supply or accelerate the availability of influenza vaccine. Within the federal government, the Department of Health and Human Services (HHS) and the Department of Defense (DOD) support the development of technologies that can be used in producing influenza vaccines. HHS's Food and Drug Administration (FDA) reviews licensing applications for new vaccine, and the Department of State is the U.S. diplomatic liaison to the international entity that declares worldwide pandemics.

GAO was asked to review federal activities for the development of alternative technologies used in producing influenza vaccine. This report examines (1) federal funding from fiscal year 2005 through March 2011 for

* This is an edited, reformatted and augmented version of a United States Government Accountability Office GAO-11-435 publication, dated June 2011.

alternative technologies and the status of manufacturers' efforts, (2) challenges to development and licensure identified by stakeholders, and (3) how HHS is addressing those challenges.

GAO reviewed HHS and DOD documents and funding data. GAO also interviewed stakeholders, including manufacturer representatives, industry associations, and other experts on challenges to development and licensure. GAO interviewed HHS officials on how they are addressing those challenges.

WHAT GAO FOUND

From fiscal year 2005 through March 2011, HHS and DOD provided about $2.1 billion in funding for the development of alternative technologies that could potentially expand the supply or accelerate the availability of influenza vaccine. Specifically, HHS and DOD have funded two alternative production technologies—cell-based and recombinant technologies, which produce vaccine in cells instead of eggs—and adjuvants, which can reduce the amount of vaccine needed to stimulate an immune response. HHS's funding supports the development of a new influenza vaccine using alternative technologies with the goal of manufacturers submitting licensing applications to FDA. DOD's funding supports the research and development of a technology that can make various vaccines, including influenza vaccines. HHS awarded $1 billion in contracts to manufacturers to develop cell-based technology, with manufacturers making progress toward licensure. HHS and DOD funded $296.5 million in contracts and $86.9 million in technology investment agreements, respectively, for the development of recombinant technology. HHS also awarded about $152 million in contracts for the development of adjuvanted influenza vaccines. Two manufacturers receiving HHS funds plan to submit licensing applications for their adjuvanted vaccines to FDA within the next 2 years.

Some stakeholders said low demand, high research and development costs, and regulatory challenges can hinder the development and licensure of new vaccines using alternative technologies. For example, despite the United States using more seasonal vaccine than any other country, some stakeholders told us that low vaccination rates can decrease incentives for manufacturers to develop new influenza vaccines using alternative technologies because there is not sufficient demand for new products. Some stakeholders said high research and development costs can also decrease manufacturers' incentives; however, HHS noted that increased investments in this area have generated a significant interest in this type of research and development. Some stakeholders also told us that some of FDA's guidance documents are not sufficiently comprehensive. FDA officials told us that their guidance documents cannot cover all possible scenarios; thus, they regularly meet with manufacturers to discuss issues and provide advice.

HHS is addressing challenges in the development and licensure of new influenza vaccines using alternative technologies. For example, HHS intends to fund the establishment of specialized facilities that will provide support and expertise to manufacturers. Additionally, through FDA, HHS plans to facilitate the review of licensing applications for new influenza vaccines using alternative technologies and to enhance FDA's staff expertise.

HHS, DOD, and the Department of State reviewed a draft of this report. In commenting on a draft of this report, HHS and DOD agreed with GAO on its findings. The Department of State did not provide comments. HHS provided suggestions to clarify the discussion.

ABBREVIATIONS

CDC	Centers for Disease Control and Prevention
DOD	Department of Defense
FDA	Food and Drug Administration
HHS	Department of Health and Human Services
NIH	National Institutes of Health
PCAST	President's Council of Advisors on Science and Technology

June 27, 2011

The Honorable Fred Upton
Chairman

The Honorable Henry A. Waxman
Ranking Member
Committee on Energy and Commerce
House of Representatives

The Honorable Bennie G. Thompson
Ranking Member
Committee on Homeland Security
House of Representatives

The Honorable Roy Blunt
United States Senate

The Honorable Joe Barton
House of Representatives

Influenza, in both its seasonal and pandemic forms, is an ongoing public health concern. Seasonal influenza may begin as early as August and generally diminishes by April in the northern hemisphere. It has been associated with 3,000 to nearly 50,000 deaths each year in the United States in recent decades, according to the Department of Health and Human Services's (HHS) Centers for Disease Control and Prevention (CDC).[1] Pandemic influenza, which periodically causes a global outbreak of serious illness with the potential for many more deaths than seasonal influenza, has occurred four times in the past 100 years.[2] In the late 1990s and early 2000s, detection of the H5N1 avian influenza (also known as "bird flu") virus in animals raised concerns among experts that it or another influenza virus might mutate into a strain that could lead to a human influenza pandemic.[3] The recent 2009 H1N1 influenza pandemic reinforced the need to be prepared for future influenza pandemics.

The federal government, specifically HHS and the Department of Defense (DOD), funds the research and development of alternative technologies that can be used in producing human influenza vaccines as a part of its pandemic influenza preparedness efforts.[4] According to HHS, HHS's and DOD's funding represents virtually all of the federal government's investment in this type of research and development. Vaccines are considered the first line of defense against seasonal and pandemic influenza, as they can prevent infection and control the spread of the disease. Furthermore, influenza vaccines are—along with diagnostic tools and treatments such as antiviral drugs—a type of medical countermeasure that can be used to protect the population during public health emergencies.[5] In 2005, HHS issued the *HHS Pandemic Influenza Plan* (Plan) for responding to an influenza pandemic.[6] One of the goals stated in the Plan is to have sufficient domestic capacity to produce enough pandemic vaccine to cover the United States' population within 6 months of a pandemic declaration.[7] These global declarations are made by the United Nations' World Health Organization, to which the Department of State is the United States' diplomatic liaison.[8] HHS also laid out its intent to support the development of new influenza vaccines using alternative technologies that could help achieve this goal. DOD plays an active role in pandemic influenza preparedness in order to maintain the military's readiness and ongoing military operations abroad, such as stockpiling antiviral drugs for use during a pandemic and developing other countermeasures.[9] In addition to ensuring the military's readiness, DOD's pandemic preparedness goals include being able to support U.S. government efforts to save lives, reduce human suffering, and slow the spread of infection.[10]

Challenges in the production of 2009 H1N1 pandemic vaccines caused fewer doses of vaccine to be available early in the pandemic than manufacturers had initially estimated; this heightened interest in the status of vaccine technologies that provide alternatives to egg-based technology. Egg-based technology is used to make all influenza vaccine currently licensed for the U.S. market by the Food and Drug Administration (FDA), the agency within HHS responsible for licensing and regulating influenza vaccines for the U.S. market. It is a well-established technology that has been in use for decades; however, it has demonstrated certain limitations in speed and efficiency in producing influenza vaccine as evidenced in the delay in producing the 2009 H1N1 pandemic vaccine supply. Given the limitations of egg-based technology and the vulnerability of chicken flocks to infectious diseases, the federal government has funded the development of alternative technologies that can be used to produce new influenza vaccines. Vaccines produced using these alternative technologies may be used during the annual influenza season or during a pandemic in order to respond faster or to create a greater supply than is possible with the current technology and production capacity. New influenza vaccines using alternative technologies are being pursued by influenza vaccine manufacturers that have egg-based influenza vaccines currently licensed for marketing and distribution in the United States or internationally, as well as by manufacturers that currently only have products in development. No influenza vaccines using alternative technologies have yet been licensed in the United States.

You asked us to review the federal government's actions regarding the research and development of alternative technologies that can be used in producing new influenza vaccines. In this report, we examine (1) federal funding from fiscal year 2005 through March 2011 in alternative technologies that can be used in producing influenza vaccines and the status of manufacturers' efforts, (2) the challenges identified by stakeholders to the development and licensure of influenza vaccines using alternative technologies, and (3) how HHS is addressing challenges to the development and licensure of influenza vaccines using alternative technologies.

To examine federal funding from fiscal year 2005 through March 2011 in alternative technologies that can be used in producing influenza vaccines and the status of manufacturers' efforts, we reviewed documents pertaining to HHS's and DOD's funding for this purpose. According to HHS, HHS's and DOD's funding represents virtually all of the federal government's investment in this type of research and development. We reviewed documents from HHS on its funding from fiscal year 2005 through March 2011. These documents included semiannual reports prepared by HHS that were submitted to Congress on the department's contracts to develop influenza vaccines using alternative technologies. We also interviewed HHS officials who oversee contracts with manufacturers to assist with the research and development of influenza vaccine for the federal government. We reviewed HHS's proposals for funding the research and development of these technologies and interviewed HHS budget officials to discuss and clarify the department's efforts. Additionally, we reviewed information from DOD on its technology investment agreements from fiscal year 2005 through fiscal year 2010. We interviewed DOD officials on the department's support of alternative technologies and the status of these development efforts. To assess the reliability of HHS's contracting data, we reviewed published data across multiple years to ensure relative consistency and interviewed knowledgeable officials to clarify questions regarding the department's funding. For DOD, we compared data on its funding provided by different sources within the department. We also asked officials about its data sources and how the department validates its data. Although we did not independently verify the information provided by HHS or DOD, based on our reviews of the data and interviews with federal officials, we concluded that these data were sufficiently reliable for the purposes of our work. Additionally, to better understand these technologies we conducted site visits to three influenza vaccine manufacturing facilities, each utilizing a different production technology, and attended national conferences on influenza vaccine research and development.

To examine challenges to the development and licensure of influenza vaccines using alternative technologies, we interviewed a judgmental sample of stakeholders, which included representatives from industry associations and manufacturers and other experts. Specifically, we interviewed 15 representatives of the vaccine industry, including those from three associations that represent pharmaceutical manufacturers—the Biotechnology Industry Organization, the International Federation of Pharmaceutical Manufacturers & Associations, and the Pharmaceutical Research and Manufacturers of America. We also interviewed officials representing 12 vaccine manufacturers—which included those manufacturers pursuing the research and development of influenza vaccines using alternative technologies, as well as those that have chosen to forgo such research and development—about the factors influencing their decisions. Of these 12 manufacturers, 8 have received funding from HHS to pursue the research and development of influenza vaccines using alternative technologies, and 1 received funds from DOD. Additionally, we interviewed a judgmental sample of 12 other experts in vaccine technology on challenges to research and development and licensure. We selected these other experts, in part, based on recommendations from an initial round of interviews with members of associations representing researchers and scientists, such as the American Society for Microbiology and the Infectious Disease Society of America. Other experts we interviewed included those from provider groups—specifically the American Academy of Pediatrics, the American Congress of Obstetricians and Gynecologists, and the American Medical Association. We interviewed representatives from these provider groups about the public's and providers' concerns about influenza vaccine safety and their understanding of alternative technologies. We also reviewed peer-reviewed journal articles and federal reports on challenges to the development and licensure of influenza vaccines using alternative technologies, including HHS's medical countermeasure review and the President's Council of Advisors on Science and Technology's (PCAST) report on influenza vaccine production.[11] We also interviewed officials representing manufacturers with influenza vaccines licensed for use in other countries and officials from the Department of State, the diplomatic liaison to the United Nations' World Health Organization—the international body that declares worldwide pandemics.

To examine how HHS is addressing challenges to the development and licensure of influenza vaccines using alternative technologies, we interviewed HHS officials on their assessments of challenges to research, development, and licensure identified by stakeholders. We also interviewed HHS officials on their efforts to address these challenges, including plans to use funds available for this purpose. Additionally, we reviewed federal documents, such as a report by FDA on its plans to improve its oversight of new products, including influenza vaccines using alternative technologies.[12]

We conducted this performance audit from March 2010 through June 2011 in accordance with generally accepted government auditing standards. Those standards require that we plan and perform the audit to obtain sufficient, appropriate evidence to provide a reasonable basis for our findings based on our audit objectives. We believe that the evidence obtained provides a reasonable basis for our findings based on our audit objectives.

Background

Influenza is a contagious respiratory illness caused by a number of different influenza virus strains and can range in severity from mild to lethal.[13] Symptoms can include cough, muscle or body aches, and fatigue. Vaccination is the primary method for preventing infection with strains of the influenza virus and controlling the disease.[14] In order for a vaccine to be most effective, it needs enough well-matched antigen to stimulate a protective immune response, antigen being the active substance in a vaccine that provides immunity by causing the body to produce protective antibodies to fight off a particular influenza strain.[15] The vaccine's antigen needs to be derived from a strain that is well-matched to a specific influenza strain—in wide circulation in humans—so that the antibodies formed in response to the vaccine protect against infection from that strain. Because multiple influenza strains are in constant circulation, seasonal vaccine is produced and administered annually to protect against the three influenza strains expected to be most prevalent that year (i.e., a trivalent vaccine). In contrast, the 2009 H1N1 pandemic vaccine was formulated to match the single pandemic-causing strain (i.e., a monovalent vaccine).

Federal Government's Role in the Research and Development of Alternative Technologies and the Licensure and Regulation of Influenza Vaccines

Within the federal government, HHS is the department responsible for leading and coordinating preparedness and medical response activities to public health emergencies, per the 2006 Pandemic and All-Hazards Preparedness Act.[16] Additionally, as the principal department for protecting the public's health, HHS is the primary department funding the research and development of influenza vaccines. HHS enters into contracts with manufacturers for the development of new influenza vaccines using alternative technologies.[17] DOD also makes some investments through its technology investment agreements for the research and development of alternative technologies that can be used in producing influenza vaccine as part of its preparedness efforts in order to maintain the military's readiness.[18] Manufacturers with which these agencies have entered into contracts or technology investment agreements include large-scale influenza vaccine manufacturers that have vaccines licensed for use in the United States and internationally as well as manufacturers that currently only have vaccines in research and development.

Table 1. Federal Government's Role in the Research and Development of Alternative Technologies and the Licensure and Regulation of Influenza Vaccines

Department	Agency
Department of Health and Human Services (HHS)	• The Biomedical Advanced Research and Development Authority within the Office of the Assistant Secretary for Preparedness and Response contracts with manufacturers for influenza vaccine research and development with the goal of anufacturers submitting licensing applications to the Food and Drug Administration (FDA) for new vaccines and establishing domestic production capacity for these new vaccines. • The National Institutes of Health supports the research and development of vaccines using alternative technologies through various activities, including conducting basic and clinical research. • FDA is responsible for the licensure and regulation of influenza vaccine—including the approval of facilities in which influenza vaccine is produced—for the U.S. market. Its responsibilities include issuing guidance for new and existing vaccines and consulting with manufacturers on the development of their new vaccines. Until FDA has approved its licensing application, no manufacturer can market its influenza vaccine in the United States.[a] Once FDA issues a license for an influenza vaccine, it continues to regulate the vaccine's production and use. For example, FDA must review and approve the seasonal vaccine annually because the influenza strains included in it frequently change from one year to the next.[b]
Department of Defense (DOD)	• The Defense Advanced Research Projects Agency within DOD funds programs focused on unique and innovative research and development efforts—including the early stage research and development of alternative technologies that can be used in producing influenza vaccines—and that accelerate the discovery and research and development of medical countermeasures, in part, through the use of novel technologies.[c]

Source: GAO analysis of HHS and DOD documents.

[a] After the HHS Secretary declares a public health emergency and under certain circumstances, FDA, as delegated by the HHS Secretary, may authorize the emergency use of licensed pharmaceutical products, such as vaccines, for unapproved uses or the emergency use of unlicensed pharmaceutical products through emergency use authorizations. See 21 U.S.C. § 360bbb-3.

[b] Each manufacturer of a U.S.-licensed influenza vaccine annually submits a supplement to its initial licensing application, noting the new influenza strains selected for a given influenza season. This same process of submitting a supplement to an existing, approved licensing application was used in the licensure of vaccine for use in the United States for the 2009 H1N1 pandemic.

[c] Medical countermeasures are drugs, biological products, or devices that treat, identify, or prevent harm from a biological or other agent that may cause a public health emergency. Medical countermeasures for use during an influenza pandemic may include vaccine, antiviral drugs, personal respirators, and influenza diagnostic tests. Antiviral drugs are medications that can prevent or reduce the severity of a viral infection, such as influenza. This report focuses on influenza vaccine.

Influenza vaccines—both seasonal and pandemic—are biological products. Within HHS, FDA is the federal agency responsible for the licensure and regulation of biological products for use in the U.S. market (see app. I for additional information on the research and development and review of licensing applications for new influenza vaccines in the United States). These responsibilities include issuing guidance for existing and new vaccines and consulting with manufacturers on the development of their new vaccines, such as on how manufacturers conduct clinical trials required for licensure of new vaccines.[19] Until FDA has approved its licensing application, no manufacturer can market its biological product in the United States.[20] Table 1 summarizes the federal government's role in the research and development of alternative technologies and the licensure and regulation of influenza vaccines.

HHS Efforts to Enhance Domestic Production Capacity to Expand the Supply or Accelerate the Availability of Influenza Vaccine

Given its responsibilities for national seasonal influenza and pandemic preparedness and response, HHS has an interest in enhancing domestic production capacity—that is, enhancing the nation's overall infrastructure for influenza vaccine production—and expanding the supply or accelerating the availability of influenza vaccine. HHS began awarding contracts to enhance domestic production capacity for the current egg-based technology as early as fiscal year 2005.[21] Since fiscal year 2005, HHS has supported a program to ensure a year-round, secure, domestic egg supply; prior to this funding, manufacturers maintained a 9-month supply of eggs—enough for production only during the influenza season without any additional capacity for emergencies, such as an influenza pandemic.

Despite HHS's initial efforts to maintain a year-round egg supply, other events have occurred that highlighted the need for HHS to increase domestic production capacity for influenza vaccine and to support the introduction of influenza vaccines produced using alternative technologies. First was the unexpected loss of almost half of the influenza vaccine supply because of potential contamination during the 2004–05 season and the reliance on two domestic influenza vaccine manufacturers to supply enough vaccine for that year.[22] Second was the recognition by HHS that one of the greatest challenges to preparing for an influenza pandemic and implementing its strategy for using vaccines was the lack of production capacity within the United States. As we noted in prior work, the lack of U.S. production capacity is cause for concern among experts because it is possible that countries without domestic production capacity will not have access to influenza vaccine in the event of a pandemic if countries where vaccine is produced prohibit the export of the pandemic vaccine until their own needs are met.[23] As a result, HHS continued its funding of egg-based technology for the production of influenza vaccine to enhance domestic production capacity using this technology. For example, in fiscal year 2007, HHS entered into contracts with two manufacturers for the retrofitting of existing domestic egg-based production facilities for the production of pandemic influenza vaccine. Some of the completed facilities were used in the 2009 H1N1 pandemic, and according to HHS, when all the retrofitting is complete, one of these facility's production capacity will double and the other will triple. Third, concerns about strains of the H5N1 virus that had reemerged in the early 2000s, and continues to cause severe infection in humans, further prompted interest in alternative technologies to egg-based technology for producing influenza vaccine.[24] Strains of the H5N1 virus have infected chicken flocks and other poultry, resulting in the culling of these flocks, raising concern that the egg supply for influenza vaccine was at risk. Thus, HHS began a more concerted effort to fund the research and development of influenza vaccines using three alternative technologies. Specifically, HHS has funded the development of vaccines using two alternative production technologies—cell-based and recombinant technologies—and vaccines using a third alternative technology—antigen-sparing technology (adjuvants).

Each of these three alternative technologies has the potential to expand the supply or accelerate the availability of both seasonal and pandemic influenza vaccines (see app. II for a description of the production process for influenza vaccine using the current, egg-based technology). Expanding the supply or accelerating the availability of influenza vaccine is particularly important when there is a perceived shortage of seasonal vaccine—when vaccine is not available and demand is highest—or during a pandemic when demand increases because of increased risk of disease and death. Expanding the supply or accelerating the availability of influenza vaccine can be done in two ways. The first is to increase the overall amount of vaccine available at the end of the production process; the second is to speed up the production process itself by, for example, reducing or eliminating step(s) in the process. Table 2 describes these three alternative technologies and their potential to expand the supply or accelerate the availability of influenza vaccines (see app. III for more information on these alternative technologies).

Table 2. Alternative Technologies and Their Potential to Expand the Supply or Accelerate the Availability of Influenza Vaccine

		Potential expansion of the supply or acceleration of the availability of influenza vaccine	
		Increase the overall amount of vaccine available	Speed up the production process
Alternative technologies	Description of technology		
Cell-based technology	technology involves a production process similar to egg-based technology. For example, as with egg-based technology, the vaccine's antigen—that is, the active substance of the vaccine that stimulates a protective immune response—is produced from the influenza virus. However, rather than using fertilized eggs as the medium for producing the influenza vaccine, cell-based technology typically uses cells infected with the influenza virus for the production of vaccine. This technology for influenza vaccines typically relies on the use of well-established cell lines, such as those originally derived from the kidney cells of monkeys or canines.	X	
Recombinant technology[a]	A second type of alternative production technology, recombinant technology uses specific protein(s) or genes from the influenza virus instead of the entire virus, as used in egg-based and cell-based technologies, as the antigen for the vaccine. This technology can use cells from mammals as the medium for producing the influenza vaccine as well as cells from other sources, such as from bacteria, yeast, insects, or plants.	X	X

Table 2. Continued

Adjuvants[b]	A type of antigen-sparing technology, adjuvants are substances that may be added to an influenza vaccine to enhance the immune response, resulting in a dose-sparing capability because less antigen is needed per dose to stimulate a protective immune response. This technology can be included with influenza vaccines made using different production technologies, such as egg-based, cell-based, or recombinant technology.	X	

Source: GAO analysis of President's Council of Advisors on Science and Technology report.

[a] The Department of Health and Human Services (HHS) refers to this technology as recombinant/molecular technology. According to HHS, this technology is also used for researching and developing a universal influenza vaccine. The National Institutes of Health, which is conducting research on a universal vaccine, defines it as a vaccine that would theoretically provide protection against any strain of influenza without needing to be updated or administered every year to protect against newly emerging annual or pandemic strains.

[b] In this report, we are referring to adjuvants made using a combination of oil and water; there are different types of adjuvants that can be used with vaccines.

HHS Funding for the Development of Influenza Vaccines Using Alternative Technologies

In fiscal year 2005, with funds available from that year's appropriation, HHS funded the research and development of an influenza vaccine produced using cell-based technology.[25]

Following the release of the Plan, numerous additional appropriations became available for the acquisition and development of pharmaceutical interventions for pandemic-related purposes, including approximately $3.2 billion dedicated for vaccines.[26] HHS has since used these funds, as well as funds available from previous appropriations, for multiyear contracts for the development of influenza vaccine using cell-based technology, recombinant technology, and adjuvants. In response to the 2009 H1N1 pandemic, Congress provided HHS with a supplemental appropriation to prepare for and respond to an influenza pandemic.[27] In addition to making $1.85 billion immediately available to HHS, the 2009 supplemental appropriation made $5.8 billion available contingent upon one or more presidential notifications to Congress.[28] In August 2010, after the 2009 H1N1 pandemic had ended, HHS notified

Congress of its plan to direct some of the remaining funds toward pandemic and related preparedness activities. Specifically, HHS proposed spending $1.98 billion in a variety of vaccine-related activities, including the development of alternative technologies, such as recombinant technology.[29] According to HHS, it also uses funding available from annual appropriations, such as its fiscal year appropriations for 2009 and 2010, for pandemic-related activities.[30]

THE FEDERAL GOVERNMENT HAS PROVIDED ABOUT $2.1 BILLION IN FUNDING FOR THE DEVELOPMENT OF ALTERNATIVE TECHNOLOGIES THAT CAN BE USED IN PRODUCING INFLUENZA VACCINES, AND MANUFACTURERS ARE DEMONSTRATING PROGRESS TOWARD LICENSURE

From fiscal year 2005 through March 2011, the federal government awarded approximately $2.1 billion in contracts and technology investment agreements for the research and development of cell-based and recombinant technologies and adjuvants, which can be used in producing influenza vaccines. Manufacturers are demonstrating progress toward licensure.

HHS Has Primarily Funded the Development of Cell-Based Technology, with Two Manufacturers Completing Clinical Trials and One Manufacturer Constructing a Domestic Facility

In fiscal year 2005, HHS awarded the most funding through contracts to manufacturers to develop cell-based technology.[31] With these funds, two manufacturers are demonstrating progress toward licensure of a vaccine by completing clinical trials required to file for licensure with FDA, and one of these two manufacturers has also constructed a domestic cell-based influenza vaccine facility. HHS awarded contracts to six manufacturers—one manufacturer in fiscal year 2005 and five manufacturers in fiscal year 2006—worth a total of approximately $1 billion for the development of an influenza vaccine produced using cell-based technology (see table 3). According to HHS, it awarded multiple contracts because it expected some attrition by manufacturers as the development of new influenza vaccines progressed. Cell-based technology has the potential to increase the overall amount of vaccine

Table 3. Department of Health and Human Services (HHS) Contracts Awarded to Manufacturers for the Research and Development of Cell-Based Influenza Vaccine, Fiscal Year 2005 through March 2011

Manufacturer	Fiscal year of award	Total obligations (in millions) [a]	Development status as of March 2011
sanofi Pasteur [b]	2005	$77.0 [c]	The manufacturer concluded that cell-based technology was not more advantageous than egg-based technology, lacked a clear path for further development, and thus chose to forgo pursuit of cell-based technology. According to HHS, it terminated this contract for the development of a cell-based influenza vaccine.
GlaxoSmithKline	2006	274.8	The manufacturer completed early-stage clinical trials of its cell-based seasonal influenza vaccine in 2009 and is currently conducting early-stage clinical trials of its cell-based, adjuvanted pandemic influenza vaccine.
Novartis Vaccines	2006	220.5	The manufacturer completed clinical trials required to file for licensure and anticipates resubmitting a licensing application for its cell-based seasonal influenza vaccine to the Food and Drug Administration (FDA) in 2011.[d]
DynPort/Baxter [e]	2006	242.3[f]	The manufacturer completed clinical trials required to file for licensure and anticipates submitting a licensing application for its cell-based seasonal influenza vaccine to FDA in 2012.
MedImmune, LLC	2006	169.5	As directed by HHS, the manufacturer halted development of its cell-based seasonal and pandemic influenza vaccine in March 2009. The manufacturer resumed development of its cell-based pandemic influenza vaccine in June 2010 and is conducting preclinical studies in animals.
Solvay Pharmaceuticals [g]	2006	48.6 [h]	The manufacturer discontinued plans for the construction of a cell-based influenza vaccine production facility in the United States because of lack of commercial viability. HHS terminated the contract for the development of a cell-based influenza vaccine in June 2009.
Total		$1032.7	

Source: GAO analysis of HHS and manufacturer data.

[a] Obligations are definite commitments that establish the legal liability of a federal agency to make payments for goods or services ordered or received, immediately or in the future. Because payments are typically made as goods or services are received, the funds listed may not have been expended. Upon termination of a contract, unexpended funds may be deobligated and, depending on the terms of their appropriation, may remain available to the agency.

[b] The policy of sanofi pasteur is to spell its name without capital letters.

[c] This amount reflects a $20 million deobligation in fiscal year 2009. A deobligation refers to the cancellation or downward adjustment of previously incurred obligations.

Table 3. Continued

[d] According to Novartis Vaccines, it submitted a licensing application for its cell-based seasonal influenza vaccine to FDA in April 2009. However, in agreement with FDA, Novartis Vaccines subsequently withdrew the application in order to incorporate efficacy data at FDA's request.

[e] HHS contracted with DynPort Vaccine Company LLC (DynPort), which collaborated with Baxter International Inc., (Baxter) to develop a seasonal and a pandemic influenza vaccine using cell-based technology. Baxter oversaw the development of the vaccine, including supporting licensure efforts for the seasonal vaccine. Baxter also oversaw the completion of clinical trials for the pandemic vaccine. DynPort managed the overall project as well as clinical trials. For the purposes of this report, we refer to this contract as DynPort/Baxter because of the collaboration between the two manufacturers.

[f] This amount includes a modification of $201.3 million made in fiscal year 2007 to the existing contract. The original contract was awarded for $41 million.

[g] Abbott Laboratories purchased Solvay Pharmaceuticals in February 2010. hThis amount reflects a $250 million deobligation in fiscal year 2009.

available at the end of the production process. As of March 2011, two of the manufacturers to which HHS had awarded contracts—DynPort Vaccine Company LLC (with Baxter International Inc.) (DynPort/Baxter)[32] and Novartis Vaccines and Diagnostics Inc. (Novartis Vaccines)—have completed clinical trials required to file for licensure with FDA. While Novartis Vaccines anticipates submitting a licensing application for its seasonal influenza vaccine using cell-based technology to FDA in 2011, DynPort/Baxter anticipates submitting its licensing application to FDA in 2012.

Additionally, GlaxoSmithKline plc (GlaxoSmithKline) is currently conducting clinical trials with its adjuvanted cell-based pandemic influenza vaccine, and MedImmune, LLC is conducting preclinical studies in animals on its cell-based pandemic influenza vaccine. The remaining two contracts with sanofi pasteur[33] and Solvay Pharmaceuticals were terminated by HHS.

In addition to the six contracts awarded for the research and development of cell-based influenza vaccine, HHS also entered into a $486.6 million contract with Novartis Vaccines in fiscal year 2009 for the construction of a cell-based influenza vaccine production facility in the United States to enhance domestic production capacity.[34] According to HHS, Novartis Vaccines completed construction of this facility in November 2009 and will have qualified the facility for producing pandemic vaccine using cell-based technology, if needed, by the end of 2011. HHS expects the new facility to provide at least 25 percent of the needed domestic production capacity for pandemic vaccine. This facility also has the capacity to produce seasonal and adjuvanted influenza vaccine as well as other biological products that use this technology for other infectious diseases.

HHS and DOD Have Funded the Research and Development of Recombinant Technology, and One Manufacturer Has Submitted a Licensing Application to FDA

In fiscal year 2009, HHS awarded contracts to manufacturers for the research and development of recombinant technology. Recombinant technology has the potential to increase the overall amount of vaccine available at the end of the production process and speed up the production process itself, in part, because unlike egg-based and cell-based technologies, it does not depend on the replication of the influenza virus for production. In fiscal year 2009, HHS entered into a $34.5 million contract with Protein Sciences Corporation (Protein Sciences) for the continued development of recombinant technology for use in producing an influenza vaccine. According to HHS, if Protein Sciences' recombinant, seasonal influenza vaccine is shown to be safe and effective through clinical trials, the contract requires the company to establish enough domestic manufacturing capacity to provide finished vaccine within 12 weeks of the beginning of a pandemic and to produce at least 50 million doses of pandemic vaccine within 6 months of the beginning of a pandemic.[35] In May 2011, HHS extended its contract with Protein Sciences for 2 years with $46.8 million of additional funding.

In February 2011, HHS awarded two additional contracts for the research and development of pandemic influenza vaccines using recombinant technology. HHS awarded contracts to Novavax, Inc. (Novavax) for $97.3 million and VaxInnate, Inc. (VaxInnate) for $117.9 million each for a 3-year period. According to HHS, if the manufacturer and department mutually agree, each respective contract may be extended for an additional 2-year period, resulting in contract amounts totaling $179.1 million for Novavax and $196.6 million for VaxInnate (see table 4).

In contrast to HHS's contract awards specifically designated for influenza vaccine described above, DOD's funding efforts have been more generally targeted toward the research and development of technologies that could be used in producing these vaccines. For example, in fiscal year 2010, DOD entered into technology investment agreements with manufacturers and research institutes—totaling approximately $86.9 million—for the research and development of recombinant technology through a DOD initiative called Blue Angel. The Blue Angel initiative is intended to accelerate ongoing programs that would potentially assist the federal government in providing a governmentwide response to an influenza pandemic.[36] Under the Blue Angel initiative, DOD supported the initial testing of a production process using recombinant technology to produce antigen—the active substance in a vaccine that stimulates the production of protective antibodies—using the 2009 H1N1 pandemic strain.[37] According to DOD, although the initiative did not result in a finished vaccine, the first batch of antigen was produced within 30 days of receiving information on the pandemic-causing strain.

Table 4. Department of Health and Human Services (HHS) Contracts Awarded to Manufacturers for the Research and Development of Recombinant Influenza Vaccine, Fiscal Year 2009 through March 2011

Manufacturer	Fiscal year of award	Total obligations (in millions) [a]	Development status as of March 2011
Protein Sciences	2009, 2011	$81.3	According to HHS, the contract requires Protein Sciences to establishenough domestic manufacturing capacity to provide finished vaccine within 12 weeks of the beginning of a pandemic and to produce at least 50 million doses of pandemic vaccine within 6 months of the beginning of a pandemic
Novavax	2011	97.3	According to HHS, the manufacturer is currently designing the clinical trials for its recombinant pandemic influenza vaccine.
VaxInnate	2011	117.9	According to HHS, the manufacturer is currently designing the clinical trials for its recombinant, pandemic influenza vaccine.
Total		$296.5	

Source: GAO analysis of HHS data.

[a] Obligations are definite commitments that establish the legal liability of a federal agency to make payments for goods or services ordered or received, immediately or in the future. Because payments are typically made as goods or services are received, the funds listed may not have been expended. Upon termination of a contract, unexpended funds may be deobligated and, depending on the terms of their appropriation, may remain available to the agency.

HHS and DOD Have Also Funded the Research and Development of Adjuvanted Influenza Vaccines, and Two Manufacturers Are Demonstrating Progress toward Licensure

Since fiscal year 2007, HHS has also awarded contracts for the research and development of an adjuvanted influenza vaccine. Adjuvants have the potential to increase the overall amount of vaccine available at the end of the production process by enhancing the immune response, thereby reducing the amount of antigen needed per vaccine dose. Two manufacturers have demonstrated progress toward licensure of their vaccines by completing clinical trials. HHS awarded three contracts totaling $152 million to GlaxoSmithKline, Novartis Vaccines, and Intercell AG for the research and development of an adjuvanted influenza vaccine (see table 5).[38] Of the three manufacturers awarded contracts, GlaxoSmithKline anticipates submitting a licensing application for its adjuvanted egg-based pandemic influenza vaccine to FDA for review in 2011, while Novartis Vaccines anticipates submitting a licensing application for its adjuvanted egg-based seasonal influenza vaccine to FDA for review in 2012. According to HHS, Intercell AG's clinical trials did not achieve the desired result and were ended.

Table 5. Department of Health and Human Services (HHS) Contracts Awarded to Manufacturers for the Research and Development of an Adjuvanted Influenza Vaccine, Fiscal Year 2007 through March 2011

Manufacturer	Fiscal year of award	Total obligations (in millions) [a]	Development status as of March 2011
GlaxoSmithKline [b]	2007, 2011	$70.2	The manufacturer completed clinical trials and anticipates submitting a licensing application to the Food and Drug Administration (FDA) for its adjuvanted egg-based pandemic influenza vaccine in 2011.
Novartis Vaccines [b]	2007	54.8	The manufacturer completed clinical trials and anticipates submitting a licensing application to FDA for its adjuvanted egg-based seasonal influenza vaccine in 2012.
Intercell AG [c]	2007	27	According to HHS, the manufacturer's clinical trials did not achieve the desired result and were ended.
Total		$152	

Source: GAO analysis of HHS and manufacturer data.

a Obligations are definite commitments that establish the legal liability of a federal agency to make payments for goods or services ordered or received, immediately or in the future. Because payments are typically made as goods or services are received, the funds listed may not have been expended. Upon termination of a contract, unexpended funds may be deobligated and, depending on the terms of their appropriation, may remain available to the agency.

b These manufacturers also have an adjuvanted cell-based pandemic influenza vaccine under development.

c HHS originally awarded the contract for adjuvant research and development to IOMAI Corporation. Because Intercell AG acquired IOMAI Corporation in August 2008, we refer to Intercell AG.

In addition to its awards through contracts with manufacturers, HHS also provided $4 million in funding to the National Institutes of Health (NIH)— an agency within HHS—for H5N1 "mix-and-match" studies starting in March 2008.[39] According to HHS, these studies are designed to determine whether the adjuvant from one manufacturer can be safely and effectively combined with the antigen from another manufacturer in the case of a public health emergency, such as an influenza pandemic.[40] The ability to combine the antigen from one manufacturer with the adjuvant from another manufacturer could increase the overall vaccine supply during a pandemic. The preliminary preclinical studies in animals with a H5N1 vaccine were completed in early 2009 in preparation for clinical testing by NIH. However, NIH delayed its work on the H5N1 vaccine to conduct clinical trials testing the unadjuvanted and mix-and-match 2009 H1N1 pandemic vaccine as part of HHS's response to the pandemic. According to NIH officials we spoke with, NIH resumed work on the H5N1 mix-andmatch studies in May 2011; officials anticipate completing clinical trials for these studies in 2012.

DOD has also funded the development of adjuvants for use with influenza vaccine. In fiscal year 2009, DOD entered into a technology investment agreement for $3.3 million with the Infectious Disease Research Institute. According to DOD, the department is currently awaiting the results of completed animal studies using an adjuvanted vaccine.

Some Stakeholders Identified Challenges to the Development And Licensure of Influenza Vaccines Using Alternative Technologies

Some stakeholders and federal reports identified three primary challenges to the development and licensure of influenza vaccines using alternative technologies: low demand, high research and development costs, and regulatory challenges.

Some Stakeholders Said Low Demand Hinders the Development of Influenza Vaccines Using Alternative Technologies

Some stakeholders told us that low demand because of low vaccination rates hinders manufacturers' willingness to develop seasonal influenza vaccines using alternative technologies.[41] According to CDC, during the 2009–10 influenza season, national vaccination rates reached an estimated 41 percent of the population aged 6 months or older for the seasonal vaccine, and an estimated 27 percent for the separate 2009 H1N1 pandemic vaccine.42 Each influenza season more vaccine is produced than is actually used, even in years where there has been a perceived shortage of influenza vaccine because of challenges in the production process. Data from CDC, FDA, and the American Medical Association confirm that—despite an increase in the total amount of influenza vaccine produced and distributed since at least 2001—more doses of seasonal vaccine are produced than distributed each year, including in years when there were few licensed manufacturers or a perceived vaccine shortage (see table 6). This excess vaccine expires and is destroyed at the season's end as it will not be useful for the next influenza season, when a new vaccine will need to be formulated using the three influenza strains expected to be most prevalent that year. Additionally, despite the increase in influenza vaccine production and distribution and the United States using more seasonal vaccine than any other country, 5 of 12 manufacturer representatives, 1 of 3 industry association representatives, and 2 of 12 other experts we interviewed said that this low demand decreases incentives for manufacturers to develop new seasonal influenza vaccines using alternative technologies.

Stakeholders told us that there are a number of reasons why demand for seasonal influenza vaccine is low. For example, two experts stated that patients commonly do not view seasonal influenza as a serious disease, and another expert and an industry association representative stated there is a need for more patient education on the safety of influenza vaccine to overcome patient and provider hesitancy. Researchers have also found that patients and providers have concerns about influenza vaccine.[43] One manufacturer representative also noted that the current influenza vaccine is less effective for certain populations, such as the elderly, which also decreases demand. We have previously reported that according to CDC, a recommendation from a physician or other health care provider is the most important factor in an individual's decision to get vaccinated.[44] Additionally, a recent review of survey data found that health care professionals were cited as one of three most important sources of information in making decisions about children's vaccines by 85 percent of parents surveyed.[45] CDC has made efforts to encourage providers to recommend vaccination to their patients. However, despite these efforts, available data suggest that getting providers to recommend vaccination for their patients has been difficult.[46] CDC told us that it is working closely with numerous partners to implement an influenza vaccine communication plan utilizing multiple forms of media to reach the general public as well as specific target populations.

HHS officials acknowledged the challenge of low demand for seasonal influenza vaccine; however, they said manufacturers remain interested in pursuing the development of new influenza vaccines using alternative technologies. For example, according to department officials, manufacturers have more than two dozen influenza vaccines in development, and many of these manufacturers have received funds from HHS.

Table 6. Number of U.S.-Licensed Manufacturers of Seasonal Influenza Vaccine and Number of Doses Produced and Distributed for the 2000–01 through 2010–11 Influenza Seasons

Influenza season	Number of licensed manufacturers	Total number of doses produced (in millions)	Total number of doses distributed (in millions)
2000–01	3	78	70
2001–02	3	88	78
2002–03	3	95	83
2003–04	3	87	83
2004–05	3[a]	61	57
2005–06	4	92	82
2006–07	5	121	104
2007-08	6	141	113
2008-09	6	143-146	111
2009-10[b]	6	114-115	114
2010-11 (est.)	6[c]	160-165	163

Source: GAO analysis of Centers for Disease Control and Prevention, Food and Drug Administration, and American Medical Association data.

Note: Table includes the number of doses produced by manufacturers and distributed to customers, such as medical supply distributors, physicians, or other types of providers.

[a] Of the three manufacturers of seasonal influenza vaccine for the 2004–05 influenza season, two produced and distributed vaccine and one ceased production and did not distribute any vaccine for the U.S. market after its license was suspended by the United Kingdom in October 2004. In addition to these three manufacturers, two foreign manufacturers' vaccines were purchased by the Department of Health and Human Services for potential use in the United States under an investigational new drug protocol; however, none of these doses were distributed.

[b] In the 2009-10 season, U.S.-licensed manufacturers also produced the 2009 H1N1 pandemic vaccine, which was purchased exclusively by the federal government for distribution in the United States. According to the Centers for Disease Control Prevention, approximately 147 million doses were available for states to order, and about 119 million were shipped to state-designated locations.

[c] The manufacturers of vaccine licensed for the 2010–11 season and their vaccines (in parentheses) were CSL Biotherapies (Afluria), GlaxoSmithKline plc (Fluarix), ID Biomedical Corporation (FluLaval), MedImmune, LLC (FluMist), Novartis Vaccines and Diagnostics, Inc. (Fluvirin and Agriflu), and sanofi pasteur (Fluzone and Fluzone High-Dose).

Some Stakeholders Said High Research and Development Costs Decrease Incentives for Developing Influenza Vaccines Using Alternative Technologies

Some stakeholders said that high research and development costs required for the development of influenza vaccines can decrease manufacturers' incentives to pursue new influenza vaccines using alternative technologies. Six of the manufacturer representatives we spoke with said that research and development costs are high. Furthermore, five manufacturer representatives we spoke with noted that clinical trials in particular contributed to high research and development costs. For example, a representative for one manufacturer we spoke with noted the significant costs associated with the research and development of its currently licensed egg-based influenza vaccine, estimating that his company has spent $400 million alone on clinical trials. One small-scale manufacturer conducting clinical trials for a new influenza vaccine using an alternative technology estimated that it spends $150,000 per day on these trials and other expenses as it moves toward applying for licensure. In addition, PCAST—a presidential advisory council—found in a recent report on influenza vaccine research and development that constructing a cell-based influenza vaccine production facility could cost more than $1 billion and it could take over 30 years to recover the investment.[47]

Access to capital is important to manufacturers because of these high research and development costs. A manufacturer representative and an industry association representative that we spoke with told us that manufacturers' difficulties in raising capital to finance research and development costs deterred or slowed the development of new influenza vaccines produced using alternative technologies. One manufacturer representative told us that in the current economic market it has been challenging for his firm to find investors. Three other manufacturer representatives noted that their decision making is also influenced by perceptions of whether the benefits of a new influenza vaccine will offset these high research and development costs by increasing production efficiency or supporting higher prices for the new product compared to the current vaccine.48 HHS told us that it has worked to address this issue through its funding for influenza vaccines using alternative technologies and that its support of manufacturers' efforts has helped to change the return on investment such that manufacturers have more incentive to pursue the development of new influenza vaccines using alternative technologies. Additionally, HHS noted that increased investments in this area have generated a significant interest in this type of research and development.

Some Stakeholders Identified Regulatory Challenges That Hinder the Development of Influenza Vaccines Using Alternative Technologies

Some stakeholders identified two regulatory challenges to the development of influenza vaccines using alternative technologies. First, some stakeholders and recent federal reports identified weaknesses in FDA's "regulatory science" capacity—that is, its ability to utilize resources, such as staff expertise, to develop new tests and measures to assess the safety, efficacy, quality, and performance of FDA-regulated products, such as influenza vaccines.[49,50] Three manufacturer representatives, one industry association representative, and three experts told us that regulatory science weaknesses at FDA create challenges in the review of new product licensing applications, including those for new influenza vaccines. In particular, stakeholders told us that FDA's staff expertise in alternative technologies affects its ability to work with manufacturers developing new influenza vaccines using these technologies, and that limited staff expertise is a challenge to efficient communication. A manufacturer representative told us that FDA's ability to conduct its own research is important in understanding the science manufacturers present in licensing applications, but noted that some of FDA's research programs have been cut in recent years thereby hindering its ability to gain needed experience. An industry association representative told us that manufacturers pursuing the development of some influenza vaccines using alternative technologies sometimes find it difficult to find FDA staff who can answer their questions. One expert said that many experienced senior leaders in FDA's biologics division—where licensing applications for new vaccines are reviewed—have left the agency in recent years; therefore, reviewers are less familiar with these alternative technologies. This expert said this lack of familiarity can make it more difficult for manufacturers to work with reviewers to explain the technology to them.

Some recent federal reports have echoed stakeholders' concerns about FDA's regulatory science capacity. According to a recent HHS report, FDA needs to be able to conduct applied research in order to better incorporate advances in life sciences research and knowledge into the regulatory process. In order to make that possible, the report states that FDA needs greater staff expertise and infrastructure.[51] In addition, a 2007 report prepared for the FDA Science Board—an FDA advisory group—found that the development of products based on new science cannot be adequately regulated by FDA because of a lack of capacity to review new technologies.[52] However, FDA officials told us that they are not aware of actual examples of lack of expertise within the agency and that their staff consists of highly qualified scientists. Furthermore, FDA officials noted the continuing education that staff members engage in to maintain their proficiency in technological advances as well as the quality of FDA's research programs. The agency said it has the scientific and regulatory experience to adequately assess the safety and effectiveness of vaccines for use in the United States, but as noted later in this report, it continues to fund improvements in regulatory science capacity and staff expertise.

Some stakeholders also identified a second challenge, namely that FDA's written guidance and consultation with manufacturers on some of the requirements for licensure of new influenza vaccines using alternative technologies is not sufficiently comprehensive.[53] They noted that FDA's guidance documents do not include all of the various scenarios manufacturers may encounter. Additionally, one manufacturer representative said it can take months to arrange a formal meeting with FDA officials. Another manufacturer representative noted that FDA often conducts its discussions with manufacturers in stages, which can limit their ability to plan for long-term issues. According to stakeholders, this lack of detail and incremental approach can hinder manufacturers' abilities to plan their research and development efforts, including those for new influenza vaccines, because they are uncertain as to what requirements they must meet in order to obtain licensure. For example, two manufacturer representatives said that it is unclear what size clinical trials will be required for influenza vaccines using alternative technologies because the guidance documents available are not specific enough in laying out these requirements. In addition, PCAST found in a recent report on influenza vaccine research and development that there is currently uncertainty about the regulatory pathway for recombinant influenza vaccines and recommended that guidance be developed on areas including criteria for formulation, safety, immunogenicity, and efficacy.[54] Also, one manufacturer representative told us that his company was repeating clinical trials for an adjuvanted vaccine that had already been performed in Europe because the company had been unaware of certain FDA requirements for data that are not typically required for similar vaccines or by regulatory authorities in other countries. The manufacturer representative noted that this situation could have been avoided if FDA had provided a more complete explanation of the requirements in this regard.

FDA officials acknowledged that its guidance documents are high level, explaining that specific instructions are unique to the product as guidance documents cannot cover all possible scenarios. In its comments, HHS officials noted that FDA's guidance is intended to provide a regulatory framework, adding that guidance cannot be specific to individual manufacturing processes because these processes are trade secrets. Because of their inability to be very specific in guidance documents, FDA officials told us that they regularly meet with manufacturers developing vaccines using alternative technologies to discuss various issues and provide advice. They also noted that the agency has a good record of achieving its goals on meeting with manufacturers within a specific time frame, adding that officials often consult with manufacturers in other ways, such as participating in teleconferences. Additionally, FDA officials said that it is necessary to consult with manufacturers in stages because their review is an iterative process. They explained that it is not always apparent what requirements may be necessary for a late phase of clinical trials because such decisions are based, in part, on results from earlier trials the manufacturer has completed. Furthermore, FDA noted that it has approved many vaccines for other diseases that used alterative technologies, such as adjuvants, and these manufacturers were able to successfully develop and license their products using FDA's guidance. Finally, FDA has published guidance on criteria for the formulation, safety, immunogenicity, and efficacy for vaccines using recombinant technology, and one manufacturer has submitted a licensing application for its influenza vaccine using this technology.55 According to HHS, part of this guidance, which is available on FDA's Web site, is related to clinical trials and is specific to clinical data needed to support the licensure of pandemic influenza vaccines.

HHS Is Addressing Challenges in the Development and Licensure of Influenza Vaccines Using Alternative Technologies

HHS has expanded its recommendations for seasonal vaccination to a larger population and has released a 10-year strategic plan to address national immunizations. HHS also plans to assist manufacturers with high research and development costs by funding the establishment of specialized facilities. In addition, HHS plans to fund the enhancement of regulatory science capacity and FDA's staff expertise to address challenges that may hinder the licensure of new influenza vaccines using alternative technologies.

HHS Has Expanded Its Vaccination Recommendations for Seasonal Influenza to a Larger Population and Has Released Its Strategy for National Immunization, Which It Expects Could Eventually Increase Demand for Vaccine

HHS has expanded its recommendations for seasonal influenza vaccination to a larger population and has released its 10-year strategy to enhance immunization rates in the United States, which it expects could eventually increase demand for influenza vaccine. In August 2010, HHS announced that it was expanding its vaccination recommendations for the 2010–11 influenza season from specific target groups based on personal risk from the disease to all persons aged 6 months and older. According to HHS, its expanded recommendations simplify the public health message to providers and to the public on who should be vaccinated against seasonal influenza. Because the 2010–11 influenza season is the first for which the recommendations are in place and the first influenza season after the 2009 H1N1 pandemic, HHS is also evaluating vaccination rates from this season for changes from previous years. For example, preliminary data from CDC suggest an increase in vaccination rates against seasonal influenza among children aged 6 months to 17 years. According to CDC, vaccination rates for this population increased by 6.7 percentage points, or from 42.3 percent during the 2009–10 influenza season to 49 percent, as of February 2011.[56] Officials noted that currently, only about 40 percent of Americans are vaccinated against seasonal influenza. HHS added that eventually demand for seasonal vaccine could increase by approximately 32 percent—or 100 million people—as a result of the expanded recommendations. Additionally, a rise in immunization rates for seasonal influenza vaccine could result in an increase in the market for this vaccine of approximately $3 billion annually, according to HHS.

In February 2011, HHS released its updated national immunization strategy, which outlines, in part, the department's efforts to address low vaccination rates for influenza.[57] This strategy, called the National Vaccine Plan, lays out HHS's efforts to enhance aspects of vaccines and vaccination rates against infectious diseases and provides a comprehensive plan for U.S. vaccine and immunization efforts from childhood to adulthood.[58] As we have noted above, several stakeholders we spoke with cited a lack of provider and public education and concerns regarding the safety of vaccines as factors affecting the demand for influenza vaccine. The National Vaccine Plan has been updated to reflect experiences from the 2009 H1N1 pandemic and describes various goals, such as enhancing provider and public education on vaccines and vaccine safety and assisting providers and the public with making informed decisions regarding vaccination. HHS also plans to develop a corresponding implementation plan that will include measurable indicators so the department can assess its progress in achieving the goals of the National Vaccine Plan; HHS anticipates releasing this implementation plan later in 2011. Additionally, HHS launched a new Web site, www.vaccines.gov in the spring of 2011 as another way of educating providers and the public on vaccines and vaccine safety.

HHS Plans to Assist Manufacturers with High Research and Development Costs by Funding the Establishment of Specialized Facilities to Provide Support and Expertise

HHS plans to assist manufacturers with high research and development costs by supporting the establishment of two or three privately owned facilities called Centers for Innovation in Advanced Development and Manufacturing that will provide support and expertise to manufacturers. HHS indicated that it intends to enter into contracts to partially fund the construction of new facilities or the retrofitting of existing facilities using approximately $478 million available from various appropriations.[59,60] Although not the primary purpose of these facilities, according to HHS, one benefit of these specialized facilities is that they could reduce smaller, less-experienced manufacturers' research and development costs by providing needed resources and knowledge about manufacturing, and reduce the technical risks of researching and developing medical countermeasures, such as influenza vaccine produced using alternative technologies. These facilities are primarily intended to provide, on a routine basis, core services that include the advanced development and manufacturing of chemical, biological, radiological, and nuclear medical countermeasures. These specialized facilities may also be used in an emergency to make pandemic influenza vaccine produced using alternative technologies, such as recombinant technology.[61] HHS noted that smaller, less-experienced manufacturers often lack the staff and other resources to address technical issues—such as those related to production, quality control, and licensure—resulting in delays and higher costs, which could cause an effort to fail. These specialized facilities would have the resources to provide manufacturers with the necessary staff, technical resources, and expertise to address these delays that can result in higher costs or effort failures.

According to HHS, these facilities might also reduce the total cost of the federal government's contracts with manufacturers. By using these specialized facilities for vaccine production, the costs associated with producing these initial vaccine doses, such as those for use in clinical trials, could be included in the facilities' operating budgets rather than in manufacturers' research and development contracts, thereby reducing the total amount of these contracts. According to HHS, the enhanced production capacity from these facilities could also help manufacturers with which HHS has contracts avoid production delays. These specialized facilities could also allow smaller, less-experienced manufacturers to focus more on developing new influenza vaccines using alternative technologies rather than on production and licensure issues. HHS anticipates awarding competitive contracts to establish these facilities in 2011 or 2012.

HHS Intends to Enhance Regulatory Science at FDA to Facilitate the Review of Licensing Applications for Influenza Vaccines Produced Using Alternative Technologies

HHS has announced plans to spend $170 million available from its fiscal year 2009 and fiscal year 2010 annual appropriations, in part, to facilitate FDA's review of licensing applications for influenza vaccines produced using alternative technologies and for other medical countermeasures.[62] Specifically, HHS intends to enhance regulatory science at FDA, that is, the development of new tests and methods to assess the safety, efficacy, quality, and performance of FDA-regulated products, such as influenza vaccines. According to HHS's report, *The Public Health Emergency Medical Countermeasures Enterprise Review*, improvements in regulatory science at FDA will help strengthen the agency's review of licensing applications.[63] In October 2010, FDA released a report outlining a proposed framework for advancing regulatory science using the funding intended by HHS for this purpose. According to FDA, improvements in regulatory science would focus on transitioning products more efficiently through review from initial concepts to licensed products. In its report, FDA identified areas in which it would focus that would potentially assist it in reviewing licensing applications for products more quickly, including during an influenza pandemic or other public health emergency.[64]

In its October 2010 report, FDA proposes additional efforts that could enhance staff expertise in reviewing licensing applications for new vaccines using alternative technologies.[65] For example, FDA intends to initiate a program to help recruit experts in emerging technologies to work as researchers and reviewers throughout the agency. FDA is also initiating the creation and support of Centers of Excellence in Regulatory Science to conduct applied regulatory science research both independently and in collaboration with the agency. According to FDA, this additional research will enhance staff expertise with emerging technologies.

FDA has issued guidance to the industry on various aspects of vaccine production, such as on the selection of cells as a medium for producing vaccines and the clinical data needed for licensure of pandemic influenza vaccines.[66] FDA officials noted that developing guidance relies on experience, which takes time to acquire, adding that they plan to continue to make themselves available to manufacturers to consult with and advise them on various aspects of the vaccine development process, including on conducting clinical trials and safety assessments.

AGENCY COMMENTS

HHS, DOD, and the Department of State reviewed a draft of this report. HHS and DOD provided written comments, which we have reprinted in appendixes IV and V, respectively. The Department of State did not provide comments. HHS also provided technical comments, which we have incorporated as appropriate.

In its comments, HHS stated that it agreed on the importance of expertise and research to the development of influenza vaccines produced using alternative technologies—cell-based and recombinant technologies and adjuvants. HHS also noted that the department has made significant contributions to advancing such expertise and research, as reflected in the collaboration within the department as well as with influenza vaccine manufacturers during the 2009 H1N1 pandemic. For example, HHS described how the Biomedical Advanced Research and Development Authority, FDA, and NIH worked with manufacturers producing both the seasonal and pandemic influenza vaccine. After approving seasonal vaccines from six manufacturers during the summer of 2009, FDA approved pandemic vaccines from four manufacturers in September 2009, and a pandemic vaccine from a fifth manufacturer in November 2009. HHS also described work done that allowed for influenza vaccine to be produced more rapidly. For example, FDA developed a technique to assess the sterility of vaccine, reducing the time for testing from 14 days to 5 days.

HHS's written comments also noted the department's concern that our description of challenges identified by stakeholders could be construed as an endorsement of them. However, as stated in our objectives, scope, and methodology, we examined challenges identified by stakeholders to the development and licensure of influenza vaccines produced using alternative technologies, and we believe our report clearly attributes these statements to the stakeholders. In response to industry concerns, HHS stated that FDA has an excellent record of responding to industry within agreed-upon time frames under applicable law and that FDA's guidance documents cannot be specific to individual manufacturing processes because these processes are trade secrets. HHS also stated that FDA provides clear guidance to manufacturers regarding the size of clinical trials and meets with sponsors of new vaccines at key stages of the product development process to provide further guidance that is informed by earlier trials.

In its comments, DOD agreed with the contents of the draft and noted that it had no substantive or administrative issues with the draft report.

We are sending copies of this report to the Secretaries of HHS, DOD, and State and to interested congressional committees. The report also is available at no charge on the GAO Web site at http://www.gao.gov.

If you or your staff have any questions about this report, please contact me at (202) 512-7114 or crossem@gao.gov. Contact points for our Offices of Congressional Relations and Public Affairs may be found on the last page of this report. GAO staff who made major contributions to this report are listed in appendix VI.

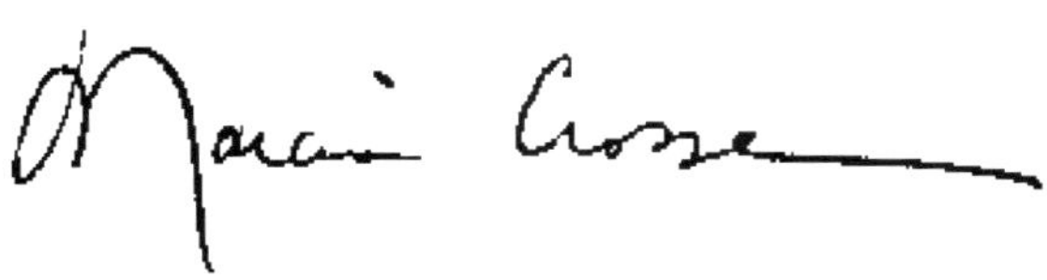

Marcia Crosse
Director, Health Care

Appendix I. The Research, Development, and Review of Licensing Applications for New Influenza Vaccine in the United States

The research, development, and review of licensing applications for new influenza vaccine for the U.S. market involve several stages.

Manufacturers producing a biological product, of which influenza vaccines are one type, must submit a licensing application for review by the Food and

Drug Administration (FDA) in order to market their vaccine in the United States. If FDA approves the application, the vaccine will be licensed for use in the United States. As shown in figure 1, this process can take, on average, a little over 10 years to complete.

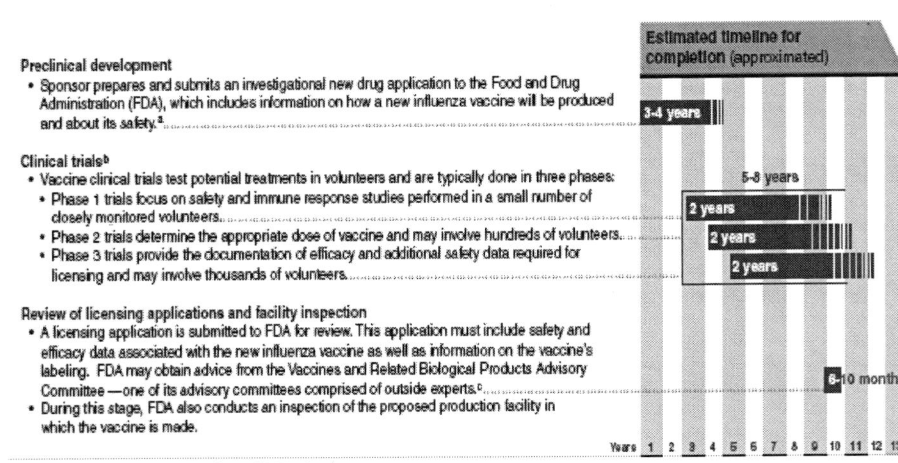

Source: GAO analysis of FDA data.

[a] A sponsor may only begin clinical trials in humans after FDA has reviewed and approved its investigational new drug application.

[b] At any time during a clinical trial, if data raise significant concerns about either safety or efficacy, FDA may request additional information or studies or may halt ongoing clinical trials.

[c] FDA's review of a licensing application generally occurs at either 6 months or 10 months after submission of a priority or a standard application, respectively.

Figure 1. Estimated Timeline for the Research, Development, and Review of Licensing Applications for New Influenza Vaccine for the United States.

APPENDIX II. INFLUENZA VACCINE PRODUCTION PROCESS USING EGG-BASED TECHNOLOGY

Both seasonal and pandemic influenza vaccines for the U.S. market are produced using egg-based technology—a complex process that involves growing seed strains in millions of fertilized chicken eggs. As shown in table 7, this process involves a sequence of steps that can take approximately 4 to 5 months to complete.

Table 7. Influenza Vaccine Production Process Using Egg-Based Technology

Step of production process	Description
Identification and selection of most prevalent strain(s)[a]	• Entities such as the United Nations' World Health Organization, the Centers for Disease Control and Prevention, and the Department of Defense conduct surveillance to identify the circulating influenza virus strain(s) expected to be most prevalent. • The Food and Drug Administration (FDA) decides which strain(s) U.S. manufacturers must include in the influenza vaccine.[b]
Development of modified strain	• One of three laboratories develops a modified strain that has the characteristics of the circulating strain(s) and grows well in eggs.[c] This step takes approximately 3 weeks to complete. • The modified strain undergoes additional testing in one of the collaborating centers associated with the United Nations' World Health Organization before being distributed to manufacturers.[d] This testing also takes approximately 3 weeks to complete.
Development, growth, and purification of seed strain	• After receiving the modified strain, manufacturers inject it into batches of fertilized chicken eggs to produce a seed strain that can be used for large-scale vaccine production. The modified strain is now called a seed strain. This process takes approximately 3 weeks to complete. • The virus seed strain is injected into millions of fertilized eggs and incubated so the strain can grow. Incubation takes approximately 2 to 3 days. • The virus is collected from the eggs and then inactivated so it is no longer infectious and is unable to cause disease.[e] • The virus is then purified and used to produce a concentrated batch of antigen—the active substance of the vaccine that stimulates the protective immune response. • Producing one batch of antigen takes approximately 2 weeks; a new batch can be started every few days.

Table 7. Continued

Testing, filling, and packaging of influenza vaccine	• Manufacturers and FDA test the vaccine using reagents produced and supplied by FDA to determine the potency, purity, and yield of the vaccine and that the potency of the antigen is sufficient to produce protective antibodies—molecules produced by a person's immune system that help fight infection.[f] This testing takes approximately 2 weeks. • Manufacturers then fill vaccine doses into vials or syringes. Labels are applied toinclude information such as the expiration date. This step takes approximately2 weeks. • FDA releases all lots of influenza vaccine and may conduct additional testing of the vaccine before officially releasing it for distribution. This additional testing occurs concurrently with the manufacturer's testing of the bulk vaccine. This testing can take up to 1 week.

Source: GAO analysis of FDA and United Nations' World Health Organization documents.

Notes: The seasonal influenza vaccine is called a trivalent vaccine because it contains three strains of the influenza virus. A pandemic vaccine, which follows the same basic production process as a seasonal vaccine, is called a monovalent vaccine because it includes only the one pandemic-causing strain.

[a] The number of influenza strains used varies depending on the type of influenza vaccine being developed. Because multiple influenza strains are in constant circulation, seasonal vaccine is produced annually to protect against the three influenza strains expected to be most prevalent that year (i.e., a trivalent vaccine). In contrast, the 2009 H1N1 pandemic vaccine was formulated to match the single pandemic-causing strain (i.e., a monovalent vaccine).

[b] FDA conducts this strain selection process in consultation with its Vaccines and Related Biological Products Advisory Committee.

[c] These three laboratories are located at CSL Biotherapies in Australia, the National Institute for Biological Standards and Control in the United Kingdom, and New York Medical College in the United States. Also, for a seasonal vaccine a modified strain is developed for each of the three influenza strains selected.

[d] This network of laboratories includes five collaborating centers associated with the United Nations' World Health Organization located in Australia, China, Japan, the United Kingdom, and the United States. The Centers for Disease Control and Prevention is the collaborating center in the United States.

[e] At this stage in the process, the virus seed strain is referred to as a virus. Additionally, unlike the injectable influenza vaccine, the live attenuated vaccine is administered as a nasal spray and does not require inactivation because of the weakened nature of the virus in the vaccine.

[f] FDA is one of the four United Nations' World Health Organization essential regulatory laboratories responsible for producing and distributing referencing agents for vaccine testing. Reagents are substances used to, for example, measure or detect components during product development. Potency tests are a measure of the vaccine's ability to stimulate an immune response. Sterility tests are intended to determine purity by detecting and identifying vaccine contaminants. Also, antibodies are molecules produced by the immune system that help fight infections.

APPENDIX III. EGG-BASED AND ALTERNATIVE TECHNOLOGIES FOR USE WITH INFLUENZA VACCINES

Both seasonal and pandemic influenza vaccines for the U.S. market are produced using egg-based technology—a complex process that involves growing seed strains in millions of fertilized chicken eggs.[1] The antigen for an egg-based influenza vaccine—the active substance in a vaccine that provides immunity by causing the body to produce protective antibodies to fight off a particular influenza strain—is derived from strains well matched to the strains in wide circulation. In order for a vaccine to be most effective, it needs to contain enough antigen to stimulate a protective immune response.[2]

Egg-Based Technology

Egg-based technology has been used to produce influenza vaccine for several decades. Department of Health and Human Services (HHS) officials we spoke with described it as a "tried and true" production technology with which regulators and manufacturers are familiar. This technology utilizes fertilized eggs as the medium for producing the vaccine.[3] Additionally, several decades of safety and efficacy data on the influenza vaccine produced using egg-based technology are available.

However, the timeliness of vaccine production is hindered, in part, by egg-based technology's reliance on seed strain development and growth. Another factor affecting the production timeline is the amount of antigen produced per egg. For example, during the 2009 H1N1 pandemic, vaccine delivery was delayed, in part, because of poorer yields of antigen per egg than expected. Also, the amount of influenza vaccine that can be produced depends on the manufacturer's egg supply. It generally takes 12 to 18 months to establish an egg supply large enough to meet the demands of either seasonal or pandemic influenza. Some experts we spoke with expressed concern that despite keeping chicken flocks producing the eggs in secure conditions to prevent contamination, these flocks are at risk of infection by, for example, the H5N1 avian influenza virus (also known as "bird flu").

Alternative Technologies for Use with Influenza Vaccines

Alternative technologies that can be used in producing influenza vaccines include alternative production technologies—such as cell-based and recombinant technologies—as well as the use of adjuvants.[4] While various alternative technologies are in development, in this report we focus on these three because these are the alternative technologies the federal government has primarily funded.

These three technologies have the potential to expand the supply or accelerate the availability of both seasonal and pandemic influenza vaccines. Expanding the supply or accelerating the availability of influenza vaccine is particularly important during times of a perceived seasonal vaccine shortage—when vaccine is not available and demand is highest— or during a pandemic when demand increases because of increased risk of disease and death. Expanding the supply or accelerating the availability of influenza vaccine can be done in two ways. The first is to increase the overall amount of vaccine available at the end of the production process; the second is to speed up the production process itself by, for example, reducing or eliminating step(s) in the process.

Cell-Based Technology

The key potential benefit to cell-based technology is the ability to increase the overall amount of vaccine available at the end of the production process. This technology for influenza vaccines typically relies on the use of well-established cell lines, such as those originally derived from the kidney cells of monkeys or canines. These cells can exponentially increase in number, allowing for the rapid expansion of the medium used for influenza vaccine production. Additionally, cells can be stored in freezers and prepared for use within days or weeks for large-scale production demands. Vaccines using cell-based technology are licensed for use in the United States for use against other infectious diseases, such as polio. Both seasonal and pandemic vaccines using such technology are also licensed in other countries, such as those in the European Union, including Germany and Spain. Cell-based seasonal and pandemic vaccines are also licensed for use in Iceland and Norway.

Despite the potential benefits of cell-based technology, there are challenges associated with its use. Similar to egg-based technology, cell-based technology relies on seed strain development and growth to obtain the influenza vaccine's antigen. For example, during the 2009 H1N1 pandemic, manufacturers had low production yields in both eggs and cells when they started vaccine production, which resulted in limited supplies for delivery to the public. Also, cell-based technology has not yet been licensed for use with influenza vaccine for the U.S. market. Additionally, few manufacturers have established domestic production capacity for influenza vaccine using this technology, and construction costs for cell-based facilities are high. For example, the construction costs for Novartis Vaccine and Diagnostics Inc.'s cell-based facility in Holly Springs, North Carolina, were over $1 billion, of which HHS funded approximately 40 percent and the manufacturer funded the remaining 60 percent.

Recombinant Technology

Recombinant technology potentially increases the overall amount of vaccine available at the end of the production process and speeds up the production process itself. First, this technology can also utilize specialized cells—from mammals or from other sources, such as from bacteria, yeast, insects, or plants—that can exponentially increase in number as the medium for influenza vaccine production, allowing for the rapid expansion of the medium used for influenza vaccine production. Recombinant technology also has the potential to speed up the production process because it does not rely on the development and growth of a seed strain to obtain the influenza vaccine's antigen. Instead, antigen is derived from the protein(s) on the surface of the influenza virus or from the virus's genes. Recombinant technology is currently used in U.S.-marketed vaccines against other diseases, such as hepatitis B and the human papillomavirus, so FDA has experience reviewing licensing applications for vaccines produced using this technology.

However, influenza vaccine using recombinant technology has not yet been licensed for use in the United States. Although some influenza vaccine has been produced for use and is currently being used in clinical trials, influenza vaccine has not yet been produced on a large scale using this production technology. One manufacturer, Protein Sciences Corporation, has submitted a licensing application to FDA for a recombinant seasonal influenza vaccine, but some experts we spoke with said it is unlikely we will know the benefits of this technology in producing influenza vaccine for several years.

Adjuvants

Adjuvants' antigen-sparing capability has the potential to increase the amount of vaccine available at the end of the production process. Adjuvants—which can be used with influenza vaccines produced using egg-based, cell-based, or recombinant technologies—can enhance the immune response, thereby reducing the amount of antigen needed per vaccine dose. By reducing the amount of antigen needed per vaccine dose, adjuvants could increase the overall influenza vaccine supply. Adjuvants have other benefits beyond potentially accelerating the delivery of influenza vaccine (see table 8).

Table 8. Additional Potential Benefits of Adjuvants

Potential benefit	Description
Enhance immune response in certain populations	Adjuvants can help enhance the immune response in certain populations that tend to respond poorly to vaccination, such as the elderly or those with underlying health conditions.
Enhance immune response	Adjuvants have the potential to enhance the immune response to protect against influenza for multiple years.
Cross protection against multiple influenza viral strains	Adjuvants, in some cases, have been found to elicit an antibody response that may be protective against similar strains of influenza viruses, thereby enhancing the potential efficacy of influenza vaccine.[a] For example, some research has shown that an adjuvanted influenza vaccine against the H5N3 strain provides protection against the H5N1 strain.[b]

Source: GAO summary of President's Council of Advisors on Science and Technology data and peer-reviewed data.

[a] An antibody is a molecule produced by the immune system that helps fight infections.

[b] See Iain Stephenson, Roberto Bugarini, Karl G. Nicholson, Audino Podda, John M. Wood, Maria C. Zambon, and Jacqueline M. Katz, "Cross-reactivity to Highly Pathogenic Avian Influenza H5N1 Viruses after Vaccination with Non-Adjuvanted and MF-59-Adjuvanted Influenza A/Duck/Singapore97 (H5N3) Vaccine: A Potential Priming Strategy," *Journal of Infectious Diseases*, no. 191 (2005): 1210-5.

Seasonal influenza vaccines administered with adjuvants are licensed for use in other countries for targeted populations, such as the elderly. Adjuvants are licensed for use with seasonal influenza vaccine in other countries, such as those in the European Union, including Belgium and Italy. Adjuvanted seasonal influenza vaccines are also licensed for use in Argentina, Columbia, Hong Kong, Mexico, the Republic of South Africa, New Zealand, and Thailand. Adjuvants were also used with the 2009 H1N1 pandemic vaccine in other countries. These other countries include Canada and Malyasia.

Although adjuvants have been used in other vaccines licensed for the U.S. market—such as in vaccine against tetanus—FDA has not approved a licensing application for a seasonal influenza vaccine using this technology in the United States; adjuvants were also not used in the U.S. supply of 2009 H1N1 pandemic vaccine. Some experts have noted potential concerns regarding the safety of repeated, annual administration of adjuvants in healthy populations—such as young adults—in a seasonal influenza vaccine.

APPENDIX IV. COMMENTS FROM THE DEPARTMENT OF HEALTH AND HUMAN SERVICES

DEPARTMENT OF HEALTH & HUMAN SERVICES — OFFICE OF THE SECRETARY

Assistant Secretary for Legislation
Washington, DC 20201

JUN 06 2011

Marcia Crosse
Director, Health Care
U.S. Government Accountability Office
441 G Street N.W.
Washington, DC 20548

Dear Ms. Crosse:

Attached are comments on the U.S. Government Accountability Office's (GAO) draft report entitled, "INFLUENZA VACCINE: Federal Investments in Alternative Technologies and Challenges to Development and Licensure" (GAO-11-435).

The Department appreciates the opportunity to review this report prior to publication.

Sincerely,

Jim R. Esquea
Assistant Secretary for Legislation

Attachment

GENERAL COMMENTS OF THE DEPARTMENT OF HEALTH AND HUMAN SERVICES (HHS) ON THE GOVERNMENT ACCOUNTABILITY OFFICE'S (GAO) DRAFT REPORT ENTITLED, "INFLUENZA VACCINE: FEDERAL INVESTMENTS IN ALTERNATIVE TECHNOLOGIES AND CHALLENGES TO DEVELOPMENT AND LICENSURE" (GAO-11-435)

The Department appreciates the opportunity to review and comment on this draft report.

Regulatory Capacity and Expertise

The Department agrees with GAO that expertise and in-house state-of-the-art research is important and critical, and we believe that we have made significant contributions to advancing such expertise and research, as described below.

The 2009-2010 influenza season was very unusual. A new and very different viral strain of influenza (2009 H1N1), was not identified as being in circulation until production of the seasonal influenza vaccines had already been initiated, and therefore, was not included in the seasonal vaccine. In response to the need, components of HHS, including the Food and Drug Administration (FDA) the Biomedical Advanced Research and Development Authority (BARDA), and the National Institutes of Health (NIH) worked collaboratively with industry, which produced both the pandemic influenza vaccine and the seasonal vaccine, to protect the public from influenza. After approving six seasonal vaccines during the summer of 2009, FDA was able to approve pandemic influenza vaccines from four manufacturers on September 15, 2009 and from a fifth manufacturer on November 10, 2009. The pandemic vaccine was a good match to the circulating pandemic virus. These outcomes reflected extensive communication and cooperation between the influenza vaccine industry and the Department.

In 2009-2011, we conducted cutting-edge scientific work that significantly improved the ability to produce influenza vaccine more rapidly. First, FDA developed a technique to assess vaccine sterility that cut the duration of the test from 14 to 5 days. Second, FDA scientists developed a more rapid way to make one of the key materials needed to test the potency of influenza vaccine. Scientists throughout HHS are currently working to develop new potency tests that would make both seasonal and pandemic influenza vaccines available more quickly. Additionally, multiple HHS agencies are advancing research on universal influenza vaccines. For example, researchers at FDA and the Centers for Disease Control and Prevention (CDC) developed and tested in mice a candidate "universal," off-the-shelf vaccine designed to reduce illness and slow the spread of disease caused by new influenza A viruses that emerge suddenly, spread quickly, and for which there is no specific vaccine available. A single dose of the vaccine reduced illness and virus levels in mice later infected with highly virulent H1N1 and H3N2 (seasonal influenza), and H5N1 (bird flu).[1] In addition, scientists at the NIH Vaccine Research Center used DNA vaccine technology in a two-step immunization approach that was effective against a diverse array of influenza virus strains in mice, ferrets, and monkeys.[2] These types of vaccine approaches, if effective in humans, could be stockpiled and then used to reduce deaths and severe illness in the event of delayed production of traditional vaccine against a newly emergent influenza virus.

[1] "Single-dose Mucosal Immunization with a Candidate Universal influenza Vaccine Provides Rapid Protection from Virulent H5N1, H3N2 and H1N1 Viruses," PLoS 2010, 5(10) October 4, http://dx.plos.org/10.1371/journal.pone.0013162.

[2] C-J Wei, *et al*. Induction of broadly neutralizing H1N1 influenza antibodies by vaccination. *Science* DOI: 10.1126/science.1192517 (2010)

GENERAL COMMENTS OF THE DEPARTMENT OF HEALTH AND HUMAN SERVICES (HHS) ON THE GOVERNMENT ACCOUNTABILITY OFFICE'S (GAO) DRAFT REPORT ENTITLED, "INFLUENZA VACCINE: FEDERAL INVESTMENTS IN ALTERNATIVE TECHNOLOGIES AND CHALLENGES TO DEVELOPMENT AND LICENSURE" (GAO-11-435)

All of these activities required working very closely with industry, foreign regulators, and other domestic public health agencies. FDA consistently provided one-on-one detailed guidance specific to issues related to each manufacturer, and to industry in general during this process. In addition, HHS increased active surveillance to monitor the safety of these vaccines as they were deployed to the public.

Responsiveness to Industry

We note that GAO includes a finding that that stakeholders GAO interviewed identified regulatory challenges that hinder the development of influenza vaccines using alternative technologies. GAO cites as the sources of this finding meetings attended, journal articles reviewed, and various stakeholders interviewed, including manufacturers pursuing alternative technologies.

Although HHS understands that GAO is simply describing the views that the stakeholders provided, with no intention of endorsing such views, restating such claims may be construed as an endorsement of them. HHS believes that it is important that GAO clarify that their intent is not to substantiate nor endorse the stakeholder views.

Some of the challenges associated with the development of influenza vaccine technologies are documented on FDA's website, including transcripts of Vaccine and Related Biological Products Advisory Committee Meetings (VRBPAC), where topics included in the GAO draft report were discussed.

- http://www.fda.gov/AdvisoryCommittees/CommitteesMeetingMaterials/BloodVaccinesandOtherBiologics/VaccinesandRelatedBiologicalProductsAdvisoryCommittee/ucm129568.htm,
- http://www.fda.gov/downloads/AdvisoryCommittees/CommitteesMeetingMaterials/BloodVaccinesandOtherBiologics/VaccinesandRelatedBiologicalProductsAdvisoryCommittee/UCM197912.pdf
- http://www.fda.gov/downloads/AdvisoryCommittees/CommitteesMeetingMaterials/BloodVaccinesandOtherBiologics/VaccinesandRelatedBiologicalProductsAdvisoryCommittee/UCM167162.pdf
- http://www.fda.gov/downloads/AdvisoryCommittees/CommitteesMeetingMaterials/BloodVaccinesandOtherBiologics/VaccinesandRelatedBiologicalProductsAdvisoryCommittee/UCM215266.pdf
- http://www.fda.gov/ohrms/dockets/ac/08/transcripts/2008-4384T1_1.htm
- http://www.fda.gov/ohrms/dockets/ac/08/transcripts/2008-4384T1_2.htm
- http://www.fda.gov/ohrms/dockets/ac/08/transcripts/2008-4384T-add.htm
- http://www.fda.gov/AdvisoryCommittees/CommitteesMeetingMaterials/BloodVaccinesandOtherBiologics/VaccinesandRelatedBiologicalProductsAdvisoryCommittee/default.htm

FDA has actively used these meetings to explore many of the challenges and issues associated with developing these new technologies.

GENERAL COMMENTS OF THE DEPARTMENT OF HEALTH AND HUMAN SERVICES (HHS) ON THE GOVERNMENT ACCOUNTABILITY OFFICE'S (GAO) DRAFT REPORT ENTITLED, "INFLUENZA VACCINE: FEDERAL INVESTMENTS IN ALTERNATIVE TECHNOLOGIES AND CHALLENGES TO DEVELOPMENT AND LICENSURE" (GAO-11-435)

In response to comments by representatives of regulated industry regarding the timeliness of agency responsiveness, the Department would also like to note that FDA adheres to timelines agreed upon with industry during the Prescription Drug User Fee Act (PDUFA) negotiations for scheduling meetings and responding to submissions. FDA regulations describe key meetings that are helpful in resolving questions and issues raised during the course of clinical development.[3] FDA has an excellent record of responding to such meeting requests.

To assist industry and when appropriate, FDA develops guidance to clarify the requirements under a given regulation. The intent of FDA's guidance documents is to provide a regulatory framework. Guidance cannot be specific to individual manufacturing processes, as these very processes are trade secrets. Therefore, FDA strongly encourages manufacturers, especially vaccine manufacturers, to meet with the agency to discuss the scientific options appropriate for their specific needs.

Regarding the clarity of requirements for clinical trials, FDA provides clear guidance to manufacturers regarding the size of clinical trials. FDA meets with the sponsors regularly as they develop their products, starting with the pre-investigational new drug (IND) phase. FDA also strongly encourages sponsors to meet with the agency at the end of phase II, which is a critical milestone in product development. The size of clinical trials will be informed by the efficacy and safety endpoints, which will depend upon the product, the clinical indication, and information gleaned during product development. In addition, FDA has issued two guidance documents that describe endpoints used for clinical trials, including one specific to clinical data needed to support the licensure of pandemic influenza vaccines. They can be found on FDA's website.[4]

---

[3] (1) pre-IND meetings (21 CFR 312.82), (2) certain end of Phase 1 meetings (21 CFR 312.82), (3) end of Phase 2/pre-Phase 3 meetings (21 CFR 312.47), and (4) pre-NDA/BLA meetings (21 CFR 312.47)

[4] http://www.fda.gov/BiologicsBloodVaccines/GuidanceComplianceRegulatoryInformation/Guidances/Vaccines/ucm074786.htm
http://www.fda.gov/BiologicsBloodVaccines/GuidanceComplianceRegulatoryInformation/Guidances/Vaccines/ucm074794.htm

APPENDIX V: COMMENTS FROM THE DEPARTMENT OF DEFENSE

THE ASSISTANT SECRETARY OF DEFENSE

1200 DEFENSE PENTAGON
WASHINGTON, DC 20301-1200

HEALTH AFFAIRS

June 3, 2011

Ms. Marcia Crosse
Director, Health Care
U.S. Government Accountability Office
441 G Street, NW
Washington, DC 20548

Dear Ms. Crosse:

This is the Department of Defense's (DoD's) response to the Government Accountability Office (GAO) Draft Report, GAO-11-435, "INFLUENZA VACCINE: Federal Investments in Alternative Technologies and Challenges to Development and Licensure," dated May 19, 2011, (GAO Code 290847). Thank you for the opportunity to review and comment.

Though the draft report does not contain any recommendations for our action, the report does contain information that adds to the DoD's knowledge base on influenza. We found no substantive or administrative issues with the draft report. If you require additional information, the points of contact on this issue are COL James Boles (Functional) and Mr. Gunther Zimmerman (Audit Liaison). COL Boles may be reached at (703) 578-8444, or James.Boles@ha.osd.mil. Mr. Zimmerman may be reached at (703) 681-4360, or Gunther.Zimmerman@tma.osd.mil.

Sincerely,

Jonathan Woodson, M.D.

APPENDIX VI. ACKNOWLEDGMENTS

Director; George Bogart; Cathleen Hamann; Mariel Lifshitz; Gay Hee Lee; John Rancourt; and Kristal Vardaman made key contributions to this report.

End Notes

[1] CDC, "Estimates of Deaths Associated with Seasonal Influenza—United States, 1976-2007," *Morbidity and Mortality Weekly Report*, vol. 59, no. 33 (2010): 1057-1062.

[2] These pandemics include the "Spanish flu" of 1918, which killed an estimated 675,000 people in the United States; the "Asian flu" of 1957, which caused approximately 70,000 deaths in the United States; the "Hong Kong flu" of 1968, which caused an estimated 34,000 deaths in the United States; and the recent 2009 H1N1 pandemic, which caused from 8,870 to 18,300 deaths in the United States. Influenza pandemics can have successive "waves" of disease and last for up to 3 years.

[3] According to the United Nations' World Health Organization, since 2003, 553 cases of human H5N1 influenza have appeared in 15 countries, resulting in a total of 323 deaths as of May 13, 2011.

[4] Alternative technologies for influenza vaccines can also be referred to as non-egg based technologies or next generation technologies. However, for this report, we use alternative technologies. Examples of these technologies include cell-based technology or adjuvants, described later in this report. Other examples include quadravalent vaccine, that is, a vaccine made using four strains of influenza virus.

[5] Medical countermeasures are drugs, biological products, or devices that treat, identify, or prevent harm from a biological and other agent that may cause a public health emergency. Medical countermeasures for use during an influenza pandemic may include vaccine, antiviral drugs, personal respirators, and influenza diagnostic tests. Antiviral drugs are medications that can prevent or reduce the severity of a viral infection, such as influenza. This report focuses on influenza vaccine.

[6] HHS, *HHS Pandemic Influenza Plan* (Washington, D.C., 2005), 24. HHS's Plan is only part of the federal government's planning efforts for responding to a pandemic. The President of the United States released two documents for a broader response: (1) the *National Strategy for Pandemic Influenza*, which provides a framework for future planning efforts for how the country will prepare for, detect, and respond to a pandemic, and (2) the *National Strategy for Pandemic Influenza Implementation Plan* (Implementation Plan), which further clarifies the roles and responsibilities of governmental and nongovernmental entities and provides preparedness guidance for all segments of society. This Implementation Plan includes 324 action items, some of which are related to enhancing domestic production capacity and supporting the development of alternative technologies for use in producing influenza vaccine.

[7] According to HHS, there was an overabundance of 2009 H1N1 pandemic vaccine available

[6] months after the declaration of the 2009 H1N1 pandemic. However, some experts we spoke with noted that the egg-based technology currently used to make influenza vaccine and the limited U.S. production capacity hindered the delivery of the 2009 H1N1 pandemic vaccine during the pandemic's peak—the time when it was most needed and in greatest demand According to CDC, the first wave of the 2009 H1N1 pandemic peaked in the United States in May and June, with a second wave peaking in October 2009. Additionally, one federal report on influenza vaccine research and development from a presidential advisory committee noted that the pandemic vaccine continued to be unavailable in sufficient quantities during the second wave of the pandemic that began in August 2009. In fact, first doses of the 2009 H1N1 pandemic vaccine did not become available until early October 2009.

[8] As part of its overall mission to protect public health, the United Nations' World Health Organization is the international entity that monitors global influenza outbreaks and declares pandemics based on the pattern of outbreaks in its regions. The *National Strategy for*

Pandemic Influenza assigned the lead for the U.S. government's diplomatic role in international efforts to address a pandemic influenza to the Department of State.

[9] The vulnerability of the U.S. armed forces to an influenza pandemic was demonstrated during World War I when at least 43,000 U.S. servicemembers died—about half of all the deaths of U.S. servicemembers during World War I—because of influenza or influenzarelated complications, and another 1 million servicemembers were hospitalized.

[10] DOD, Office of the Assistant Secretary of Defense, *Department of Defense Implementation Plan for Pandemic Influenza* (Washington, D.C., 2006). 11HHS, *The Public Health Emergency Medical Countermeasures Enterprise Review* (Washington, D.C., 2010), and PCAST, *Report to the President on Reengineering the Influenza Vaccine Production Enterprise to Meet the Challenges of Pandemic Influenza* (Washington, D.C., 2010).

[12] FDA, *A Framework for FDA's Regulatory Science Initiative: Advancing Regulatory Science for Public Health* (Washington, D.C., 2010).

[13] There are three types of influenza viruses: A, B, and C. However, only influenza A viruses cause pandemics. Influenza A viruses are further categorized into subtypes according to differences in the outer surfaces of the virus. These influenza A subtypes are further characterized into strains, which can mutate, or change genetically, over time. Small mutations result in seasonal or common influenza; more substantial changes can result in a pandemic.

[14] Vaccination is one part of a multilayered prevention strategy against influenza that also includes treatment with antiviral drugs and nonpharmaceutical countermeasures, such as regular hand washing and social distancing actions.

[15] Antibodies are molecules produced by the immune system that help fight infections.

[16] Pub. L. No. 109-417, § 101, 120 Stat. 2831, 2832. Public health emergencies may include influenza pandemics.

[17] According to HHS, the National Institutes of Health (NIH) has a history of supporting the research and development of alternative technologies for use in producing influenza vaccine. For example, as early as 2000, NIH awarded $4.93 million in grants to three manufacturers for the research and development of influenza vaccines using alternative technologies. In addition to supporting the testing of influenza vaccines using alternative technologies in preclinical studies in animals and clinical trials, NIH has supported many collaborative projects with academia and industry. These projects have an emphasis on applied research and early stage assessment of new and improved technologies for influenza vaccines, such as the use of adjuvants, and evaluating alternative vaccine technologies, such as recombinant technology. According to NIH officials, the agency's efforts are intended to further scientific knowledge and to provide services and expertise to enable the translation of new technological ideas into products which benefit public health.

[18] The Defense Advanced Research Projects Agency within DOD enters into and funds these technology investment agreements. A technology investment agreement is a type of financial assistance instrument meant to increase the involvement of commercial firms in the department's research, development, and demonstration programs. Technology investment agreements are not considered contracts, cooperative agreements, or grants. *See* 10 U.S.C. § 2371(a).

[19] Clinical trials are used to test the safety and efficacy of potential treatments in human volunteers. They occur in multiple phases, which vary based on the size and objective of the study. Studies range in size from a small number of closely monitored volunteers to thousands of volunteers. In most cases, before clinical trials can be conducted in human volunteers, researchers conduct preclinical studies in animals.

[20] However, after the HHS Secretary declares a public health emergency and under certain circumstances, FDA, as delegated by the HHS Secretary, may authorize the emergency use of licensed pharmaceutical products, such as vaccines, for unapproved uses or the emergency use of unlicensed pharmaceutical products through emergency use authorizations. *See* 21 U.S.C. § 360bbb-3.

[21] Egg-based technology is a complex process that involves growing seed strains in millions of fertilized chicken eggs. This process involves a sequence of steps that can take approximately 4 to 5 months to complete. Egg-based technology is used to produce both seasonal and pandemic influenza vaccines for the U.S. market.

[22] GAO, *Influenza Vaccine: Shortages in 2004–05 Season Underscore Need for Better Preparation*, GAO-05-984 (Washington, D.C.: Sept. 30, 2005), 1.

[23] GAO, *Influenza Pandemic: Efforts Under Way to Address Constraints on Using Antivirals and Vaccines to Forestall a Pandemic*, GAO-08-92 (Washington, D.C.: Dec. 21, 2007), 26. This situation occurred during the 2009 H1N1 pandemic when CSL Biotherapies in Australia and GlaxoSmithKline, plc in Canada were required to fulfill their domestic orders for the pandemic vaccine prior to releasing vaccine to the United States.

[24] Human infections from strains of the H5N1 virus first occurred in 1997 in Hong Kong, Special Administrative Region.

[25] *See* Consolidated Appropriations Act, 2005, Pub. L. No. 108-447, 118 Stat. 2809, 3112, 3138. During this fiscal year, other appropriations were also available for the acquisition and development of pharmaceutical interventions for pandemic-related purposes, including vaccines. *See* Consolidated Appropriations Act, 2004, Pub. L. No. 108-199, 118 Stat. 3, 251, and Emergency Supplemental Appropriations Act for Defense, the Global War on Terror, and Tsunami Relief 2005, Pub. L. No. 109-13, 119 Stat. 231, 276, 280. Many of these appropriations are available without fiscal year limitation.

[26] *See* Departments of Labor, Health and Human Services, and Education, and Related Agencies Appropriations Act, 2006, Pub. L. No. 109-149, 119 Stat. 2833, 2857; Department of Defense, Emergency Supplemental Appropriations to Address Hurricanes in the Gulf of Mexico, and Pandemic Influenza Act, 2006, Pub. L. No. 109-148, 119 Stat. 2680, 2783, 2786; Emergency Supplemental Appropriations Act for Defense, the Global War on Terror and Hurricane Recovery, 2006, Pub. L. No. 109-234, 120 Stat. 479; and Revised Continuing Appropriations Resolution, 2007, Pub. L. No. 110-5, 121 Stat. 8, 33. Many of these appropriations are available without fiscal year limitation.

[27] Supplemental Appropriations Act, 2009, Pub. L. No. 111-32, 123 Stat. 1859, 1884-86.

[28] Each such presidential notification must designate amounts as emergency funds required to address critical needs related to emerging influenza viruses.

[29] HHS, *Amended Spending Plan for 2009 Supplemental Funding* (Washington, D.C., 2010), as reported to Congress in August 2010. According to HHS, the amended spending plan will provide funding for further development of medical countermeasures as recommended in *The Public Health Emergency Medical Countermeasures Review*.

[30] *See* Departments of Labor, Health and Human Services, and Education, and Related Agencies Appropriations Act, 2009, Pub. L. No. 111-8, 123 Stat. 524, 779, and Departments of Labor, Health and Human Services, and Education, and Related Agencies Appropriations Act, 2009, Pub. L. No. 111-117, 123 Stat. 3034, 3255. Portions of these appropriations are available without fiscal year limitation.

[31] According to HHS, the required criteria for manufacturers to receive this funding were (1) develop cell-based influenza vaccine technology, (2) obtain FDA licensure of cell-based influenza vaccine, and (3) construct a domestic cell-based influenza vaccine facility.

[32] HHS contracted with DynPort Vaccine Company LLC (DynPort), which collaborated with Baxter International Inc. (Baxter) to develop a seasonal and a pandemic influenza vaccine using cell-based technology. Baxter oversaw the development of the vaccine, including supporting licensure efforts for the seasonal vaccine. Baxter also oversaw the completion of clinical trials for the pandemic vaccine. DynPort managed the overall project as well as clinical trials. For the purposes of this report, we refer to this contract as DynPort/Baxter because of the collaboration between the two manufacturers.

[33] The policy of sanofi pasteur is to spell its name without capital letters.

[34] According to HHS, HHS and Novartis Vaccines shared the cost of the construction of the new production facility, with HHS funding approximately 40 percent of the total cost and Novartis Vaccines funding the remaining 60 percent.

[35] In April 2008, prior to entering into this contract with HHS, Protein Sciences submitted a licensing application to FDA for its seasonal recombinant influenza vaccine which, as of March 2011, was still under review. According to a Protein Sciences official, FDA is expected to complete its review this year.

[36] DOD also provides funding through its Blue Angel initiative to other entities, such as universities and other federal agencies.

[37] This testing was done through DOD's Accelerated Manufacture of Pharmaceuticals program, one of the programs included in DOD's Blue Angel initiative. This program focuses on the creation of a production process capable of making 3 million doses of any vaccine, including influenza vaccine, within 12 weeks of identifying a particular microbe. Under this program, DOD entered into contracts with manufacturers totaling approximately $51.6 million. Because the Accelerated Manufacture of Pharmaceuticals program is not specific to influenza, we did not include it when determining the amount of federal investments made for the research and development of alternative technologies for use in producing influenza vaccines.

[38] HHS awarded the contract for adjuvant research and development to IOMAI Corporation. Because Intercell AG acquired IOMAI Corporation in August 2008, we refer to Intercell AG.

[39] The Biomedical Advanced Research and Development Authority within HHS's Office of the Assistant Secretary for Preparedness and Response provided this funding through an interagency agreement with NIH for the mix-and-match studies. The Biomedical Advanced Research and Development Authority coordinates the development and procurement of medical countermeasures for public health emergencies. The National Institute of Allergy and Infectious Diseases, within NIH, is conducting this research. This institute also supports other research related to influenza, including providing research resources to help develop influenza vaccine candidates and supporting projects focusing on routes of vaccine administration.

[40] Typically, the same manufacturer produces both the antigen and the adjuvant to be used together in the vaccine.

[41] The challenge of low demand and subsequent discussions of challenges associated with high research and development costs and regulatory challenges do not refer to times when there is an ongoing pandemic, during which demand may increase because of increased risk of disease and death.

[42] CDC, *Final Estimates for 2009–10 Seasonal Influenza and Influenza A (H1N1) 2009 Monovalent Vaccination Coverage – United States, August 2009 through May 2010* (Atlanta, Ga.: 2010). CDC acknowledges that its survey-based estimates of seasonal vaccination rates for the 2009–10 season are overestimates since the projected number of persons receiving seasonal influenza vaccination exceeds the number of doses distributed in the United States. However, CDC notes that these estimates are consistent with previously published interim estimates.

[43] For example, see Pritish K. Tosh, Thomas G. Boyce, and Gregory A. Poland, "Flu Myths: Dispelling the Myths Associated with Live Attenuated Influenza Vaccine," *Mayo Clinic Proceedings*, no. 83 (2008): 77-84. Also, see Deborah A. Gust, Natalie Darling, Allison Kennedy, and Ben Schwartz, "Parents with Doubts About Vaccines: Which Vaccines and Why," *Pediatrics*, no. 122 (2008): 718-725.

[44] GAO, *Influenza Vaccine: Issues Related to Production, Distribution, and Public Health Messages*, GAO-08-27 (Washington, D.C.: Oct. 31, 2007), 40.

[45] The other two most important sources for parents cited by respondents were family members (46 percent) and friends (22 percent). Allison Kennedy, Katherine LaVail, Glen Nowak, Michelle Basket, and Sarah Landry, "Confidence about Vaccines in the United States: Understanding Parents' Perceptions," *Health Affairs*, vol. 30, no. 6 (2011): 1151-59.

[46] For example, a 2008 phone survey of adults conducted by the National Foundation for Infectious Diseases found that almost 40 percent of respondents reported that they had never discussed influenza vaccination with their physician or other health care worker. National Foundation for Infectious Diseases, *National Consumer Survey: Doctors and Patients Not Talking Enough About Influenza Vaccination* (Bethesda, Md., September 2008).

[47] PCAST, *Report to the President on Reengineering the Influenza Vaccine Production Enterprise.*

[48] Two manufacturer representatives we spoke with noted that the current egg-based influenza vaccine is a low-profit product. According to one report we reviewed, the profit margin of the seasonal influenza vaccine is estimated to be about 20 percent, compared with the 50 percent to 95 percent profit margins that are typical in the pharmaceutical market, with highest margins for novel, proprietary drugs. PCAST, *Report to the President on Reengineering the Influenza Vaccine Production Enterprise.*

[49] Regulatory science is a term used by FDA and others to refer to the tests and measures that are used to assess the safety, efficacy, quality, and performance of FDA-regulated products.

[50] FDA Science Board, *FDA Science and Mission at Risk: Report of the Subcommittee on Science and Technology*, a special report prepared at the request of FDA (Washington, D.C., 2007); HHS, *Medical Countermeasures Enterprise Review*; PCAST, *Report to the President on Reengineering the Influenza Vaccine Production Enterprise*; and the Institute of Medicine, *Building a National Framework for the Establishment of Regulatory Science for Drug Development: Workshop Summary* (Washington, D.C., 2010).

[51] HHS, *Medical Countermeasures Enterprise Review.*

[52] FDA Science Board, *FDA Science and Mission at Risk.*

[53] According to FDA, officials consult with manufacturers through meetings, which can include technical and regulatory meetings on the pathway to licensure for their specific products. FDA officials said they also provide feedback to manufacturers during advisory committee meetings. Advisory committees, composed of outside experts, provide scientific and medical advice to FDA on the safety, effectiveness, and appropriate use of certain products. In this context, they provide a forum for public discussion of issues that may benefit manufacturers in developing new products.

[54] PCAST, *Report to the President on Reengineering the Influenza Vaccine Production Enterprise.*

[55] FDA, *Guidance for Industry: Clinical Data Needed to Support the Licensure of Seasonal Inactivated Influenza Vaccines* (Rockville, Md., May 2007), and *Guidance for Industry: Clinical Data Needed to Support the Licensure of Pandemic Influenza Vaccines* (Rockville, Md., May 2007).

[56] CDC, "Interim Results: State-Specific Influenza Vaccination Coverage – United States, August 2010-February 2011," *Morbidity and Mortality Weekly Report*, vol. 60, no. 22 (2011): 737-43.

[57] The National Vaccine Program Office is specifically leading this effort. The National Vaccine Program Office is the office within HHS's Office of the Assistant Secretary for Health that coordinates the federal government's vaccine- and immunization-related activities.

[58] HHS, *2010 National Vaccine Plan: Protecting the Nation's Health through Immunization,* (Washington, D.C., 2010).

[59] *See* Pub. L. No. 109 -148, 119 Stat. 2786; Pub. L. No. 109-234, 119 Stat.479; Pub. L. No. 111-32, 123 Stat. 1884; Pub. L. No. 111-8, 123 Stat. 779; Pub. L. No. 111-17, 123 Stat. 3255. Many of these appropriations are available without fiscal year limitation.

[60] Contracts entered into for this purpose will limit the government contribution for the construction of new facilities to 49 percent, with private entities contributing the remaining 51 percent. For the retrofitting of existing facilities, HHS's maximum contribution would be 75 percent, with private entities contributing the remaining 25 percent.

[61] A mandatory criterion for eligibility under the HHS contract solicitation (solicitation #11-100-SOL-00011) is that an offeror provide evidence of a commitment to supply plans for producing finished pandemic influenza vaccine within 12 weeks of receipt of a virus strain and 50 million doses within 4 months of strain receipt.

[62] *See* The Department of Defense and Full-Year Continuing Appropriations Act, 2011, Pub. L. No. 112-10, § 1835, 125 Stat. 38, 162.

[63] HHS, *Medical Countermeasures Enterprise Review.*

[64] FDA, *Regulatory Science Initiative Framework.*

[65] FDA, *Regulatory Science Initiative Framework.*

[66] FDA, *Guidance for Industry: Characterization and Qualification of Cell Substrates and Other Biological Materials Used in the Production of Viral Vaccines for Infectious Disease Indications* (Rockville, Md., February 2010), and *Guidance: Clinical Data of Pandemic Influenza Vaccines.*

End Notes for Appendix III

[1] There are two types of influenza vaccine approved for use in the United States: (1) an inactivated virus vaccine injected into muscle and (2) a live attenuated vaccine, which contains weakened influenza viruses and is administered as a nasal spray. Also, a modified viral strain is developed from the circulating virus strain. Influenza vaccine manufacturers optimize the growth of this modified strain, which is called a seed strain. This seed strain is used to produce antigen—the active substance of the vaccine that stimulates a protective immune response—and is then collected and purified.

[2] The vaccine's antigen needs to be derived from a strain that is well matched to a specific influenza strain—in wide circulation in humans—so that the antibodies formed in response to the vaccine protect against infection. Antibodies are molecules produced by the immune system that help fight infections.

[3] Producing these fertilized eggs is more difficult than producing eggs for human consumption. The fertilized eggs are typically 9 to 12 days old, and FDA requires that these eggs meet particular sanitation and other requirements.

[4] HHS refers to this technology as recombinant/molecular technology. According to HHS, this technology is also used for researching and developing a universal influenza vaccine. The National Institutes of Health, which is conducting research on a universal vaccine, defines it as a vaccine that would theoretically provide protection against any strain of influenza without

needing to be updated or administered every year to protect against newly emerging annual or pandemic strains. Also, in this report, we are referring to adjuvants made using a combination of oil and water; there are different types of adjuvants that can be used with vaccines.

INDEX

D

E

P

Q

R

S

T

U

V

W

Y